AUTONOMY & PATERNALISM

ETHICAL PERSPECTIVES MONOGRAPH SERIES

5

Autonomy & Paternalism

Reflections on the Theory and Practice of Health Care

Editors

Thomas Nys
Yvonne Denier
Toon Vandevelde

PEETERS
LEUVEN – PARIS – DUDLEY, MA
2007

A CIP record for this book is available from the Library of Congress.

ISBN-13   978-90-429-1880-1
D. 2007 / 0602 / 33

© 2007, Peeters – Bondgenotenlaan 153 – B-3000 Leuven – Belgium

TABLE OF CONTENTS

INTRODUCTION

Thomas Nys, Yvonne Denier, Toon Vandevelde

This book starts from the assumption that there is a tension between the value of autonomy and the praxis of paternalism. This seems to be a reasonable assumption: many of us share the intuition that autonomy has to do with freedom and independence, while paternalism usually involves coercion and restriction.[1] Moreover, the fact that we perceive of both concepts as enemy notions is due to historical processes. The way in which we are familiar with the term 'autonomy' was strongly influenced by a discourse of anti-paternalism. As such, the recent emphasis on autonomy is a product of the 1960s and 1970s; it is the offspring of turbulent times in which various groups reacted against practices in which people were 'spoken for' instead of being allowed to make their own choices. Women, racial minorities, homosexuals, children, patients, etc., they were all treated paternalistically, that is, as if they were not capable of living their own lives.[2] Sometimes this implied that people were kept out of harm's way at the

---

[1] The tension between autonomy and paternalism is well-documented in the literature. See, for instance, L. MAY, 'Paternalism and Self-Interest' in *Journal of Value Inquiry* 14(1980), pp. 195-216; D.N. HUSAK, 'Paternalism and Autonomy' in *Philosophy and Public Affairs* 10(1980)1, pp. 27-46; S. LEE, 'On the Justification of Paternalism' in *Social Theory and Practice* 7(1981)2, pp. 193-203; E.P. BRANDON, 'Rationality and Paternalism' in *Philosophy* 57(1982), pp. 533-536; P. HOBSON, 'Another Look at Paternalism' in *Journal of Applied Philosophy* 1(1984)2, pp. 293-304; J.C. CALLAHAN, 'Paternalism and Voluntariness' in *Canadian Journal of Philosophy* 16(1986)2, pp. 199-220; E.D. COHEN, 'Paternalism that does not Restrict Individuality: Criteria and Applications' in *Social Theory and Practice* 12(1986)3, pp. 309-335; G. DWORKIN, *The Theory and Practice of Autonomy*, Cambridge, Cambridge University Press, 1988; D. ARCHARD, 'Paternalism Defined' in *Analysis* 50(1990)1, pp. 36-42; D. ARCHARD, 'Self-Justifying Paternalism' in *Journal of Value Inquiry* 27(1993), pp. 341-352; J. KULTGEN, 'Consent and the Justification of Paternalism' in *The Southern Journal of Philosophy* 30(1992)3, pp. 89-113.

[2] For a more detailed account of these historical social processes, see A.I. TAUBER, 'Historical and Philosophical Reflections on Patient Autonomy' in *Health Care Analysis* 9(2001), pp. 299-319.

cost of belittlement or even disgrace. At other times however, the 'paternalistic' intervention even seemed to go against the general and laudable goal of protecting a person's well-being. Instead, the interference involved a misconception of personal welfare. The general public was confronted with numerous scandals which revealed that the choices which were made for the individual had serious detrimental effects on the well-being of these persons.[3] The conception of the good that was forced down these people's throats did not, in fact, do them any good. Those who claimed to know better, made some serious and irreversible mistakes which were downright inhumane. What such an attitude of 'paternalism' neglected was that a person's well-being could come in different shapes and that the best way to contribute to the welfare of individuals was to listen to them and allow them to make their own decisions. As a result, the claims of these various groups were often formulated in terms of individual rights. Most importantly, they claimed that individuals should have the right to self-determination; people should be allowed a 'space of their own' in which they could determine and pursue their own conception of the good. They should be permitted to live their own life, and this, in turn, implied that they should be respected in their autonomy conceived as the capacity for independence, personal reflection and critical decision-making. The fact that human beings are capable, at least to a certain extent, of distancing themselves from their environment, from their desires and beliefs, is intimately connected with their sense of dignity. Therefore, whenever this capacity is seriously denied or ignored, the person is not treated with appropriate respect, and instances of paternalism are obvious cases where such respect is wanting. Or so the argument goes.

Although these historical processes which have contributed to the importance of autonomy have deeply pervaded the whole of society, we focus in this book on the context of biomedical ethics. In this specific context, one often refers to the 'triumph of autonomy'. This means that within the set of ethical considerations that should be taken into account in medical decision-making, the principle of respect for autonomy has become dominant. It is believed to override

---

[3] O. O'NEILL, *Autonomy and Trust in Bioethics*, Cambridge, Cambridge University Press, 2002, pp. 14-16. According to O'Neill, it is the attention which was paid to these scandals (e.g., due to excessive media coverage) which has caused a crisis of trust in bioethics.

these other considerations or principles.[4] For example, in Beauchamp and Childress's *Principles of Biomedical Ethics*, we find the idea of an ethics based on four fundamental principles: non-maleficence, beneficence, justice, and autonomy. The triumph of autonomy suggests that these other principles have been pushed into the background and that, if there are conflicts between the demands of these principles, respect for autonomy should prevail. This implies that a traditional conception of medicine which totally revolved around the principle of beneficence and in which 'doctor knew best', was replaced by a patient-centred account. Traditional medicine was paternalistic through-and-through: its goal was to restore or promote the patient's well-being where the doctor's expertise made him the best judge regarding this conception of well-being. He knew what it took to make a patient better. The triumph of autonomy implies that we look at this traditional approach with utmost suspicion. Why should doctors know any better? If anything, we believe that doctor and patient should meet each other as equals.[5] Moreover, we also believe that there is no single correct and universal answer to the question of what constitutes a 'good life'. Hence a doctor has no right whatsoever to impose his conception of the good. In sum, our deeply rooted intuitions about equality and pluralism rally against the image of traditional and paternalist medicine.

As we noted at the outset, this book takes the triumph of autonomy and the corresponding suspicion towards paternalism as a point of departure. This is, however, only a starting point. In general, the contributors to this volume are highly critical of the triumph of autonomy and many of them question whether a sharp dichotomy between autonomy and paternalism should not be avoided in favour of a different, more adequate conception of what good medical care actually means. Before we come to these attempts to reconsider the relation-

---

[4] "For better or for worse [...] autonomy has emerged as the most powerful principle in American bioethics, the basis of much theory and much regulation, and has become the 'default principle' [...] Indisputably [...] patient autonomy has become the most powerful principle in ethical decision making in American medicine." P.R. WOLPE, 'The Triumph of Autonomy in American Bioethics' in R. DEVRIES & J. SUBEDI (eds.), *Bioethics an Society: Constructing the Ethical Enterprise*, New Jersey, Prentice Hall, pp. 38-59.

[5] It is claimed, for example, that the doctor is not the only expert involved, but that the patient has some expertise as well. For some literature on the 'expert patient', see the special issue of *Medicine, Health Care and Philosophy* 8(2005)2, pp. 147-178.

ship between autonomy and paternalism, let us look at these notions in very general terms so as to provide a conceptual framework which could serve as a background for further investigation.

1. Autonomy

Obviously, the term autonomy was not invented in the 1960s and 1970s. Its origin can be traced back to Ancient Greece where it was used to denote the privilege of city states to issue their own laws independently from the so-called 'mother nation'. The idea of independence is still paramount in contemporary conceptions of autonomy, but it is clear that its primary use no longer involves city states or nations (although it is still used in that way). Instead, we talk about the autonomy of persons. This contemporary usage of the term is often attributed to Kant, but this is a rather unfortunate interpretation because Kant conceives of autonomy as a capacity of practical reason and, as such, he is more concerned with the autonomy of moral precepts — i.e. their independence from contingent and external goals — as he is with the autonomy of individuals.

1.1 The Kantian Heritage

According to Kant, morality can only be grounded in the autonomy of the will. A Categorical Imperative, that is to say, an unconditional and universal command, can only be founded on a will which could somehow be 'a law to itself'. As long as moral precepts are based on external goals, i.e. on realizing some 'goods', they presuppose a certain interest in these goals and, as such, they remain utterly contingent. However, if morality should be grounded in autonomy, then the will should be able to operate independently from 'alienating causes'. This leads to Kant's (in)famous idea of the human person as a citizen of two worlds: an inhabitant of both a phenomenal and a noumenal realm. However, such a split between two worlds (and especially the idea of a noumenal realm *behind* or *beyond* the world of phenomena), seems to be based on a dubious metaphysics. Hence, if autonomy indeed presupposes the existence of these two worlds, then the concept rests on shaky grounds. Still, many contemporary scholars are inclined to say that the idea of the autonomy of the will still makes sense without this solution in terms of a 'two worlds' distinction.[6] Alternatively they opt for a 'two standpoints' interpretation: from an external perspective, man is subject to the laws of cause and effect, but from an internal perspective he enjoys practical freedom; i.e. he must consider himself free and unbound. According to these authors, practical freedom is the cornerstone of autonomy.

Yet, Kant's conception of autonomy is problematic for a different reason as well. It has lost its appeal because of its intimate connection with morality. Autonomy indeed means self-governance, but for Kant the emphasis is on 'governance' and not on 'self'.[7] Kant's theory is not about different individuals living their lives according to their own, personal laws. Instead, it is about the will's capacity — even in imperfect beings as ourselves — to be subjected to universal moral precepts. In fact, the contemporary idea of the individual who should be respected in his choices or preferences is quite antithetical to the Kantian idea of respect for autonomy for it would imply that we should honour a person's inclinations or *Neigungen*.

However, we should note that a huge part of the contemporary debate is still framed in a Kantian vocabulary. For example, the idea of human dignity — i.e. the principle that people should not be treated as mere means to ends — is often invoked.[8] Human beings possess a certain inviolability because they have the capacity to set ends for themselves. In this regard, many authors refer to Kant as an important source of the recent emphasis on personal autonomy. Therefore, it is important to be aware of both the similarities and the dissimilarities between our present-day conception of autonomy and its Kantian origin.

---

[6] Th. HILL, 'Kant's Argument for the Rationality of Moral Conduct' in P. GUYER (ed.), *Kant's Groundwork of the Metaphysics of Morals: Critical Essays*, Lanham, Lowman & Littlefield, 1998, pp. 249-272; O. O'NEILL, *Bounds of Justice*, Cambridge, Cambridge University Press, 2000, p. 45; Th. HILL, *Human Welfare and Human Worth: Kantian Perspectives*, Oxford, Oxford University Press, 2002, pp. 35-36; Ch. KORSGAARD, 'Kant's Analysis of Obligation' in P. GUYER (ed.), *Kant's Groundwork of the Metaphysics of Morals: Critical Essays*, Lanham, Lowman & Littlefield, 1998, pp. 62-63.

[7] O. O'NEILL, *Autonomy and Trust in Bioethics*, pp. 85-86.

[8] For a comparison between two senses of dignity — one which is inspired by Kant and another which is based on a contemporary conception of autonomy — see D. PULLMAN, 'Dying with Dignity and the Death of Dignity' in *Health Law Journal* 4(1996), pp. 197-219.

An author like Onora O'Neill, for example, stresses the dissimilarities.[9] She emphasizes that the recent celebration of autonomy is a far cry from what Kant originally meant by it. Nowadays, we stand in awe for a conception which is no longer worthy of our applause because, in neglecting its Kantian meaning, autonomy's value has faded as well. According to O'Neill the triumph of autonomy is a sad mistake; it is a typical case of 'the emperor's new clothes' where everybody refuses to acknowledge that what we celebrate is only a very scantily clad version of what actually deserves our admiration.

A return to Kant's robust conception of autonomy would reveal that autonomy is intimately linked to moral precepts like the (perfect) duties of non-coercion and non-deception. Respect for autonomy means respect for these moral principles. If so, then a return to this robust conception might enable us to overcome a contemporary malaise in biomedicine: the erosion of trust. Medicine has become a matter of contract because the recipients of care are suspicious with regard to those who should provide their services. Detailed contracts should prevent doctors from doing things their own way. However, ever more fine print in contracts has not restored trust. Much to the contrary: it has only encouraged a sphere of distrust. Instead, O'Neill's plea for robust autonomy which emphasizes unconditional adherence to moral principles is trust-increasing. Moreover, a focus on Kantian autonomy would also imply that autonomy should be respected on both sides: both doctors and patients should adhere to these moral principles. Most importantly, this entails that patients cannot take hostage of their doctors and demand from them that they satisfy their every whim or desire.

1.2 Mill's Influence

If we should look for a historical forefather of our contemporary conception of autonomy, then John Stuart Mill seems to fit that description rather well. Although Mill never uses the term 'autonomy', his plea for individual freedom in *On Liberty* is very much in line with what we consider to be the main argument for autonomy. According

---

[9] For another emphasis on the dissimilarities, see T. MEULENBERGS & P. SCHOTSMANS, 'The Sanctity of Autonomy?' in P. SCHOTSMANS & T. MEULENBERGS (eds.), *Euthanasia and Palliative Care in the Low Countries*, Leuven, Peeters, 2005, pp. 122-125; A.I. TAUBER, 'Historical and Philosophical Reflections on Patient Autonomy', p. 307.

to Mill, people should be allowed to conduct various experiments in living because a person's "own mode of laying out his existence is the best, not because it is the best in itself, but because it is his own mode".[10] Individuality (or, as we should say, autonomy) is a necessary ingredient of human well-being and this enables Mill to defend the value of self-determination on utilitarian grounds. In the name of happiness and well-being, society should promote the expression of individuality.

An individual's pursuit of personal well-being should only be curtailed by "one very simple principle" which is typically referred to as Mill's harm-principle. This principle states that the only legitimate cause for interference with a person's freedom of conduct is harm to others.[11] Put differently: harm to self is never a sufficient condition. As such Mill's theory seems to dovetail very well with the recent triumph of autonomy: we should not in any way force people to become happy in a manner that does not correspond to their own conception of the good as long as there is no other party injured or harmed.

This very simple principle, however, turns out to be notoriously difficult to interpret.[12] For example, a lot depends on the difficult and sometimes tiresome question of what is to be considered as 'harm'. It goes without saying that as long as there is disagreement about the limits of harm, there will be disagreement about the limits of the harm principle as well. However, it has been noted that the recent emphasis on the principle of autonomy has rendered medical decision-making a question of bargaining instead of an applying ethical standards to concrete situations (in a top-down fashion).[13] As such, the contours of harm need not be fixed: it is sufficient that all parties agree with a certain practice — i.e. that they consent to whatever 'harm' is done — for it to be justified. Hence the theoretical difficulties concerning the harm-principle could be settled on a pragmatic level.

---

[10] J.S. MILL, *On Liberty*, ed. M. WARNOCK, Malden, MA, Blackwell Publishing, 2003, p. 141.

[11] *Ibid.*, pp. 94-95.

[12] For some other difficulties with the harm principle, see A. WERTHEIMER, 'Victimless Crimes' in *Ethics* 87(1977)4, pp. 302-318; N. HOLTUG, 'The Harm Principle' in *Ethical Theory and Moral Practice* 5(2002), pp. 357-389.

[13] T. ENGELHARDT, *The Foundations of Bioethics*, 2nd edition, Oxford, Oxford University Press, 1998, p. 68.

Although Mill's influence on the recent debate concerning autonomy and paternalism is very obvious, it should be noted that there is an aspect which was crucial for Mill, but which is almost completely absent in the contemporary context. Apart from the claim that autonomy is necessary for personal happiness, Mill's argument in *On Liberty* is driven by a concern for moral progress. His main enemy in that respect was a growing tendency for conformism. People were prone to imitate the acts and beliefs of others and they were less concerned about whether what they believed was actually true. As such, human life was reduced to an endless repetition of the same-old-same-old without any opportunity for improvement. In order to break free from the deadlock of conformism, Mill urged to open up a space for discussion so that new ideas could be brought before the 'altar of reason'. This however implied that the experiments in living which he so vehemently defended should be able to serve in rational argumentation. And this, it should be noted, is a serious restriction. For example, Mill did not defend freedom of speech, but the freedom of thought and discussion which indicates that his primary goal was to encourage rational dialogue, that is, to compare different opinions and conceptions of the good, in order to learn from such a comparison and enable us to move forward.[14]

Both these strands in Mill — his plea for diversity and his concern for truth — do not fit easily together and they have contributed to his reputation for being a confused and muddled thinker. Apart from issues of consistency, however, it is safe to say that we no longer share his (optimist) nineteenth century faith in rationality and moral progress. Instead we celebrate the principle of respect for autonomy as a token of the limits of rationality, i.e. as way of dealing with incommensurable conceptions of the good. As such, it is a device for allowing us to live side-by-side, not a means to move forward as a whole (as a group, or community, or society). Hence, although Mill can be conceived as the godfather of our modern discourse in favour of respect for personal autonomy, his conception of individuality was framed in a context which was very different from the one in which we find ourselves today.

---

[14] See, for instance, R. VERNON, 'John Stuart Mill and Pornography: Beyond the Harm Principle' in *Ethics* 106(1996)3, pp. 622-623; J. RILEY, 'J.S. Mill's Doctrine of Freedom of Expression' in *Utilitas* 17(2005)2, p. 151; T. NYS, 'The Tacit Concept of Competence in J.S. Mill's On Liberty' in *South African Journal of Philosophy* 25(2006)4, pp. 305-328.

Still, an important idea which we inherited from Mill is that a person's right to self-determination should be restricted by conditions of competence. He leaves no doubt about it that his harm principle does not apply to children, fools and societies which should be considered in a state of 'nonage'.[15] He excludes those who are unable to take proper care of themselves, or, as he puts it, those who are incapable "of being improved by free and equal discussion". In contrast to Kant who conceived of autonomy as a metaphysical property of the will, Mill's concept of autonomy depends upon certain (mental or psychological) capacities which a person can possess in various degrees.[16]

1.3 Procedural and Hierarchical Conceptions of Autonomy

Roughly speaking we could say that, from Kant to Mill, the concept of autonomy has evolved from a term which was originally intended to express the possibility of ethical principles which were independent from contingent goals, to a notion which denotes the capacity of human beings to live their lives according to their own ideas about the good. Put differently, there was a shift from moral autonomy to personal autonomy.[17]

We could however still discern a further shift, i.e. a further restriction in scope, so to speak, from the autonomy of persons to the autonomy of desires, decisions, or choices. On these later accounts, autonomy is no longer a general or global capacity which allows individuals to exercise control over their own lives, but it essentially denotes a property of certain mental aspects of the individual. Some desires are autonomous, while others are not. Consequently, some choices — the ones that are the result of autonomous desires — bear the mark of autonomy, while others do not. In this regard, the principle of respect for autonomy implies that we should respect an individual's autonomous choices insofar as he is competent and his choices do not entail harm to others.

---

[15] J.S. MILL, *On Liberty*, p. 95.

[16] Th. HILL, 'The Kantian Concept of Autonomy' in J. CHRISTMAN (ed.), *The Inner Citadel: Essays on Individual Autonomy*, New York, Oxford University Press, 1989, pp. 91-108.

[17] For a clear presentation of the differences between both notions, see J. WALDRON, 'Moral Autonomy and Personal Autonomy' in J. CHRISTMAN & J. ANDERSON (eds.), *Autonomy and the Challenges to Liberalism*, Cambridge, Cambridge University Press, 2005, pp. 307-329.

Such more restricted accounts are influenced by authors like Harry Frankfurt and Gerald Dworkin who both employ a hierarchical conception of autonomy. According to Frankfurt, a certain desire X is autonomous if it is supported by a corresponding second-order volition Y, that is, if a person *wants* to be moved by desire X.[18] For example, my desire to take another piece of delicious chocolate cake is autonomous only if I want to be motivated by this desire (e.g., if I am not on a diet). Put differently, autonomy requires that I *identify* with the desire which moves me to action.

Although their accounts are quite similar, Dworkin puts more emphasis on the *formation* of second-order desires, that is to say, on the fact that such desires are the outcome of a process of critical reflection.[19] Critical reflection enables a person to distance himself from his first-order desires and to decide whether or not to endorse them. For example, we are all moved by envy or spite from time to time, but most of us do not identify with these 'baser' inclinations and therefore we believe that we would be better off without them. This implies that whenever we are moved by such desires, we feel that, in some way, we are moved against our will; i.e. that our desires govern us instead of the other way around. The most obvious examples of such alienating desires are cases of addiction or compulsion where the unwilling addict or neurotic is reduced to a 'passive bystander': he is led by desires with which he does not identify.

The important feature is that these theories of autonomy focus on desires. Although neither Dworkin nor Frankfurt are concerned with the principle of respect for autonomy, we should note that such respect is often framed in terms of desires or choices as well. To treat a patient with respect means that one respects his autonomous decisions. Hence, it is no longer about a person being able to exercise control over his life in general, but about honouring individual and specific choices.

In this regard, the practice of *informed consent* has become extremely important. Almost every decision in health care — certainly in the American context — should be justified by a patient's informed consent. As such, respect for autonomy has been reformulated in terms

---

[18] H. FRANKFURT, *The Importance of What We Care About*, Cambridge, Cambridge University Press, 1988, pp. 13-14.

[19] G. DWORKIN, *The Theory and Practice of Autonomy*, Cambridge, Cambridge University Press, 1988, p. 20.

of respect for a person's consent. Put differently: the triumph of autonomy is actually the triumph of the principle of informed consent. And indeed this principle seems very important: e.g., the ability to withhold their consent gives patients the right to refuse treatment, and this is a vital tool against zealous and ruthless paternalism. This basic right to nod 'yes' or 'no' seems very appropriate in a context in which people are weak and vulnerable. As such, it is a minimal instrument for the suffering individual to be heard.[20]

However, those who oppose to this restriction, argue that the practice of informed consent is far too limited in scope. On the one hand, it could prevent caretakers from administering good care (the absence of consent might be an obstacle) and, on the other hand, it could justify them in doing things which go against the individual's best interests (consent might easily be obtained and justify treatment which is actually sub-optimal). Moreover, the focus on — or should we say 'obsession with' — informed consent implies that patients are literally stalked with consent forms since each and every decision seems to require their approval. This entails that a lot of responsibility is piled upon the frail shoulders of the patient. Consequently, they might be forced to choose while they would rather rely on the judgment of experts. In this sense, it seems that patients are sometimes 'sold out' to their autonomy.[21]

1.4 The Principles of Biomedical Ethics

A theory which, in many respects, exemplifies the shift from moral autonomy to the autonomy of choices is Beauchamp and Childress's principalism. Respect for autonomy, which is one of the four principles on which their theory is based, implies respect for the autonomous choices of competent patients. Beauchamp, however, reacts against the hierarchical theories of Dworkin and Frankfurt. One of his criticisms is that a supporting second-order desire can be the result of a person having a certain first-order desire. For example, a person's will to carry on smoking, that is, to endorse his craving for a cigarette, may itself be the result of his addiction. To overcome these

---

[20] O. O'NEILL, *Autonomy and Trust in Bioethics*, p. 49.
[21] E.H. LOEWY, 'In Defense of Paternalism' in *Theoretical Medicine and Bioethics* 26(2005), pp. 445-468.

difficulties, Beauchamp maintains that the focus should shift to autonomous actions, i.e. actions which are performed (1) voluntary, (2) intentionally, and (3) with sufficient understanding.[22]

Throughout the subsequent editions of the *Principles of Biomedical Ethics*, the principle of respect for autonomy has gained in importance. Consequently, many people believe that Beauchamp and Childress have contributed to the recent 'triumph of autonomy' in medical ethics.[23] Still, it is important to emphasize that Beauchamp and Childress explicitly acknowledge that instances of paternalism can sometimes be fully justified; sometimes the other principles — beneficence, non-maleficence, and justice — should override our concern for a patient's autonomy.[24] Hence, although respect for autonomous choices is very important, it is not that important that it should outweigh all other moral considerations.

2. Paternalism

Now let us turn to the concept of paternalism. As was the case with autonomy, consensus on what paternalism means is very hard to find. To stick with the discussion of Beauchamp and Childress, they define paternalism as "the intentional overriding of a person's known preferences or actions by another person, where the person who overrides justifies the action by the goal of benefiting or avoiding harm to the person whose will is overridden".[25] This implies that non-intentional paternalism is a non-starter and that one cannot behave paternalistically if one is not aware of a person's preferences (e.g., when someone has passed out, or is unconscious, or in a coma). Moreover, paternalism entails that the interference is done with the distinct purpose of "benefiting or avoiding harm" to the individual who is interfered with. This is important, because a lot of actions which we tend to call 'paternalistic' do not, in fact, fit this description. Sometimes the intentions of the person who intervenes are aimed at avoiding

[22] T.L. BEAUCHAMP & J.F. CHILDRESS, *Principles of Biomedical Ethics*, 5th edition, New York, Oxford University Press, 2001, p. 59.

[23] T. MEULENBERGS & P. SCHOTSMANS, 'The Sanctity of Autonomy?', pp. 122-124.

[24] T.L. BEAUCHAMP & J.F. CHILDRESS, *Principles of Biomedical Ethics*, 4th edition, New York, Oxford University Press, 1994, p. 181.

[25] T.L. BEAUCHAMP & J.F. CHILDRESS, *Principles of Biomedical Ethics*, 5th edition New York, Oxford University Press, 2001, p. 178.

harm to others, or even to prevent harm to himself.[26] We might force alcoholics and drug addicts to sober up in various institutions where they are kept against their will, with the goal of cleaning the streets of such unstable individuals (because they scare us, or annoy us, or whatever), and not because it is for their own good. Admittedly, we often have mixed motives for interfering with a person's liberty of action (so-called 'impure paternalism'). Yet, what is clear though, is that interference which is not in any way based upon a concern for a person's well-being cannot be labelled paternalistic.

Another influential definition is offered by Bertrand Gert and Charles Culver.[27] They argue that instances of paternalism need not interfere with a person's liberty of action. A man who hides his wife's sleeping pills does not obstruct her freedom, but he still behaves paternalistically because he violates a moral rule; he goes behind her back and so, in a way, he deceives her. David Archard has raised some objections against this definition. According to him, what is necessary is that the paternalist has the intention of interfering with a person's opportunities for choice, and he can do so without violating any moral rule.[28]

A question which is of special interest to our topic is whether paternalism necessary entails an offence against a person's autonomy. This seems reasonable in light of the evidence that instances of paternalism are often objected to by referring to a person's right to self-determination. Yet, in the paradigm case of paternalism — a parent's behaviour towards his children — there does not seem to be a violation of autonomy since (young) children are considered incompetent. Paradoxically, cases of justified paternalism do not seem to be genuine cases of paternalism. Soft paternalism, for example, does not appear to be real paternalism. As Joel Feinberg defines it, soft paternalism is interference with a person's actions in order to make sure that the act is voluntary.[29] If we stop a person from crossing a bridge which we know is very unstable and bound to collapse, then we are justified in doing so to the extent that we believe that this person wants to cross

---

[26] J. FEINBERG, *Harm to Self: The Moral Limits of the Criminal Law*, Oxford, Oxford University Press, 1986, p. 4.

[27] B. GERT & Ch. CULVER, 'Paternalistic Behavior' in *Philosophy and Public Affairs* 6(1976)1, pp. 45-57.

[28] D. ARCHARD, 'Paternalism Defined' in *Analysis* 50(1990)1, p. 36.

[29] J. FEINBERG, *Harm to Self*, p. 12.

this bridge safely and that he does not want to plummet into the water. Yet in such cases we do not go against a person's true wishes. Much to the contrary, we want to make sure what these wishes are so as to prevent serious mistakes.

The fact that these kinds of interference do not strike us as genuine paternalism is probably the result of our everyday conception of paternalism which is strongly coloured by negative, normative associations. We believe that paternalism is wrong insofar as it treats adult, competent persons *as if* they were children[30], i.e. as if they were incompetent and unable to make choices which fit their own, well-considered conception of the good. Hence we focus on *hard paternalism*: interference with a person's liberty of action for his own good even if this goes against his voluntary, intentional, and well-informed choices.[31] A morally neutral definition needs to include the 'good' as well as the 'bad' instances of paternalism. One way of doing this is by arguing that justified cases of paternalism — although they might interfere with a person's liberty of action, or his expressed choices, or the opportunities which are available to him — do not violate his autonomy.

3. Beyond Autonomy and Paternalism? Two Strategies

In the previous paragraphs we have only sketched the concepts of autonomy and paternalism in most general terms. As said before, the contributors to this volume are highly critical with regard to the recent triumph of autonomy. However, they are critical of paternalism as well and they would not want us to return to a type of medicine which is based on the pre-1960s model. In this regard it is interesting to see that there are different ways of meeting both these demands.

First, one might believe that we should balance the value of autonomy with that of beneficence or good care. This is a conflict model. However, one might object that it is doubtful that the concept of beneficence still has any meaning outside of, or independent from, the principle of respect for autonomy. Could one do good for a patient if this implies going against his true wishes? Isn't that a contradiction?

---

[30] J. FEINBERG, *Harm to Self*, p. 5.
[31] *Ibid.*, p. 12.

Does 'the good' not lie in the eye of the beholder? Put otherwise: is there such a thing as an 'objective good'; something the individual — even in his autonomous choices — can be mistaken about? Is there some basic conception of the good we can force upon him? If not, then the idea of balancing autonomy with beneficence becomes nonsensical; or better: it is turned into a conflict which is bound to be won by the first.

A second strategy is to try and overcome the sharp dichotomy between autonomy and paternalism and to move beyond the alleged incompatibility. This strategy is to attack the concept and value of autonomy itself (and to do the same with the concept of paternalism). Hence it is claimed that respect for autonomy — although it is central in our society as a value that should be respected by our political and legal institutions — it is ill-suited for the context of health care. In fact, what a focus on autonomy ignores, with its emphasis on independence and self-sufficiency, is that people are essentially dependent beings. A feature which becomes especially apparent in a context where people are quite literally thrown upon their limits; a context in which they are ill and in need of care. In this regard it is utterly remarkable that respect for autonomy plays such a dominant role in medical ethics; a domain where there is at times very little autonomy to be respected. Moreover, according to these authors, care should not be conflated with paternalism, because good care is the product of a dialogue. The doctor or caretaker should listen to his patients even if they are unable to utter their preferences; he should be attentive to their silent voice. Obviously, this is not a conflict model, but a model of dialogue and reconciliation where doctor and patient are oriented towards the same goal: the patient's well-being.

4. The Arguments in this Volume

The various chapters of this book shed a light on different aspects of the relationship between autonomy and paternalism. Moreover, they try to conceive of how a crude tension between both concepts can be avoided. How can we do justice to an individual's personal conception of the good while, at the same time, be able to administer good care?

George Agich proposes to re-conceptualize autonomy in order to meet the demands of long-term care. Most of our contemporary conceptions of autonomy are ill-adapted to this context as they tend to focus on decisions while decisions do not play a very prominent role in everyday life. This however, does not imply that we lack autonomy if we do not pause and reflect upon our actions. It just shows that there is a more mundane sense of autonomy which is largely neglected. Therefore, Agich emphasizes the importance of *actual autonomy* (a term borrowed from Onora O'Neill) which signifies this tacit, beneath-the-surface dimension of autonomy. Respect for actual autonomy means that we recognise the individual as a socially-embedded person with a specific personality that deserves to be respected. This implies that the relation between the caretaker and the recipient of care should be dialogical and that care should be tailored to the specifics of the individual's life. Respect for actual autonomy means that care-takers should be sensitive to what the recipients deem meaningful in life. They need to focus on what we could call 'small autonomy', i.e. on the day-to-day activities which are important to an individual. They need to look for those aspects which make life worthwhile for a person. This sensitivity tends to get lost in a general account of what respect for autonomy means, that is, an account which uses autonomy merely as a justificatory tool ("keep your distance", or "do as the patient autonomously decides").

Eva Kittay makes a similar point. She argues that the demands which are posited by popular conceptions of autonomy are often too demanding. In that respect: "it seems odd that autonomy has come to command centre stage in biomedical ethics, that is, in an ethics developed for a context where individuals are especially vulnerable and unusually dependent on others for the care and expertise that can determine their continued existence and well-being". Even when the concept is attenuated to the requirement of informed consent, such consent is often "only a pale shadow of the autonomy that it is meant to embody". Moreover, it excludes people who are incapable of understanding the relevant information or who are unable to communicate their preferences. In order to overcome these problems, Kittay seeks to dissolve the sharp dichotomy and conflict between autonomy and paternalism (cf. the second strategy). The dichotomy hinges upon a distinction between the autonomous and the non-autonomous: on a divide between the competent and the incompetent. This unduly restricts the principle of respect for autonomy. Secondly, a mere focus on whether persons are treated paternalistically or respected in their autonomy ignores the larger setting in which these questions arise. As an alternative to this myopic vision on autonomy (and paternalism) Kittay defends what she calls the *caring transparent self*: "a self accommodating to the wants of another; that is, a self that defers or brackets its own needs in order to provide for another's".[32] Such a caring self is able to respect the agency that is left in those who fail to meet the present day requirements of autonomy.

Eric Matthews also has reservations with regard to the principle of autonomy. More precisely: he is doubtful whether the principle is of any use in the context of psychiatry. He agrees with Kittay that a large subset of the people who are in need of medical attention seem to lack autonomy, and hence, that it cannot be respected. Matthews traces our modern conception of respect for autonomy to Mill, but he notes that the liberty which Mill so vehemently defended only holds for a specific kind of choices: it is the freedom to make rational choices in a context where there is no rational best to decide between them (e.g., market choices). According to Matthews, it is questionable whether the choices which are presumably protected by our contemporary understanding of respect for patient autonomy could be defended on Millian grounds. There are some principles in health care which have an 'objective character', that is, which should be acknowledged by every rational person. Personal preferences or choices which endanger these principles should not be honoured out-of-hand, but they should be perceived with elevated awareness. In the context of psychiatry it may occur that patients, no matter how hard doctors try to set up a dialogue, refuse to accept treatment which, according to objective and shared standards, is in their best interests. The bottom-line of Matthews' paper is that respect for human dignity sometimes requires that we go against a person's expressed wishes or preferences (i.e. that we should go against their autonomy). As such, Matthews puts strong emphasis on rationality and its relation to human dignity. Yet, at the same time, he warns us that we should be extremely cautious because some seemingly irrational decisions may turn out to be reasonable after all. This calls for a 'sensitive exploration' of the reasons which support a patient's decisions.

David Archard focuses on the practice of informed consent as it is regarded "a specification of the principle of respect for individual autonomy". He questions whether this principle implies that we

---

[32] E.F. KITTAY, *Love's Labor: Essays on Women, Dependency and Equality*, New York, Routledge, 1999.

should obtain informed consent for every medical intervention. Archard interprets autonomy as "the capacity of individuals to govern themselves, [i.e.] to determine the direction of their lives". Therefore, he concludes that this capacity is not vitiated by the mere absence of informed consent in cases when the intervention does not preclude the individual's ability to live his life according to his own lights. A simple mouth swab, for example, leaves a person's autonomy entirely intact. Hence, if we do think that such a mouth swab is in need of serious justification, then such justification should be based on a different principle. Archard then considers *privacy* and *self-ownership* as possible arguments in favour of informed consent and he argues that neither of these values can be reduced to a more primitive principle of autonomy.[33]

Yvonne Denier addresses the connection between autonomy, physical well-being, and the 'good life' within the context of medical decision-making. According to Denier, physical well-being and considerations about 'the good' are different aspects of autonomy. She proposes a model of solidarity in which the physician is the expert concerning the objective well-being of the patient, while at the same time, the patient is the best judge regarding what is in his best interests and properly serves his own conception of the good. Like Kittay, she underscores the fact that people are essentially dependent beings, yet she also emphasizes that autonomy — i.e. independence — is something we highly value. In order to do justice to these 'ambiguities of care' we need to develop what Denier calls *careful solidarity*, that is, "the art of caring without humiliating".

Thomas Nys reconsiders the dichotomy between autonomy and paternalism. Whereas both concepts are frequently regarded as enemy notions, he argues that instances of paternalism often only make sense if they are interpreted as expressions of autonomy. The paternalist acts upon a concern for the other person's well-being and this motive often depends upon the fact that there is also something at stake for him: he is personally invested in the well-being of the cared-about object. Autonomy is then expressed outwardly, that is, in desires which involve the things he cares about. The paradoxical result is that respect for autonomy could imply that we should respect instances of paternalism. Therefore, if we value individual autonomy,

---

[33] For a related argument, see J.S. TAYLOR, 'Autonomy and Informed Consent: A Much Misunderstood Relationship' in *Journal of Value Inquiry* 38(2004), pp. 383-391.

then we should respect it on both sides: i.e. on that of the cared-about individual (the patient) as well as on that of the caretaker (the doctor). Hence, the principle of respect for autonomy is insufficient to deal with ethical problems in medical decision-making. Instead we should move to a discussion on what constitutes the good life.

Heike Smidt-Felzmann points our attention to the problem of paternalism within the setting of psychotherapy. Although early psychoanalysis was already aware of the danger of a therapist imposing his values upon the patient, this awareness proves to be insufficient to safeguard psychotherapy from the pitfalls of paternalism. However, the instruments with which we analyse the problem in ordinary health care (e.g., informed consent, coercion, deception) are too blunt and need to become more attuned to the specific context of psychotherapy. The dangers of paternalism are more subtle here (i.e. "hidden forms of influence"). For example, psychotherapy is seldom value-free, nor is it an interaction between equals. In order to attenuate the potential danger of paternalism, therapists need to make their values transparent; they need to make clear when their authority shifts from descriptive expertise to moral counselling.

References

ARCHARD, D., 'Paternalism Defined' in *Analysis* 50(1990)1, pp. 36-42.

ARCHARD, D., 'Self-Justifying Paternalism' in *Journal of Value Inquiry* 27(1993), pp. 341-352.

BEAUCHAMP, T.L. & J.F. CHILDRESS, *Principles of Biomedical Ethics*, 4th edition, New York, Oxford University Press, 1994.

BEAUCHAMP, T.L. & J.F. CHILDRESS, *Principles of Biomedical Ethics*, 5th edition, New York, Oxford University Press, 2001.

BRANDON, E.P., 'Rationality and Paternalism' in *Philosophy* 57(1982), pp. 533-536.

CALLAHAN, J.C., 'Paternalism and Voluntariness' in *Canadian Journal of Philosophy* 16(1986)2, pp. 199-220.

COHEN, E.D., 'Paternalism that does not Restrict Individuality: Criteria and Applications' in *Social Theory and Practice* 12(1986)3, pp. 309-335.

DWORKIN, G., *The Theory and Practice of Autonomy*, Cambridge, Cambridge University Press, 1988.

ENGELHARDT, T., *The Foundations of Bioethics*, 2nd edition, Oxford, Oxford University Press, 1998.

FEINBERG, J., *Harm to Self: The Moral Limits of the Criminal Law*, Oxford, Oxford University Press, 1986.

FRANKFURT, H., *The Importance of What We Care About*, Cambridge, Cambridge University Press, 1988.

GERT, B. & Ch. CULVER, 'Paternalistic Behavior' in *Philosophy and Public Affairs* 6(1976)1, pp. 45-57.

HILL, Th., 'The Kantian Concept of Autonomy', in J. CHRISTMAN (ed.), *The Inner Citadel: Essays on Individual Autonomy*, New York, Oxford University Press, 1989, pp. 91-108.

HILL, Th., 'Kant's Argument for the Rationality of Moral Conduct' in P. GUYER (ed.), *Kant's Groundwork of the Metaphysics of Morals: Critical Essays*, Lanham, Lowman & Littlefield, 1998, pp. 249-272.

HILL, Th., *Human Welfare and Human Worth: Kantian Perspectives*, Oxford, Oxford University Press, 2002.

HOBSON, P., 'Another Look at Paternalism' in *Journal of Applied Philosophy* 1(1984)2, pp. 293-30.

HOLTUG, N., 'The Harm Principle' in *Ethical Theory and Moral Practice* 5(2002), pp. 357-389.

HUSAK, D.N., 'Paternalism and Autonomy' in *Philosophy and Public Affairs* 10(1980)1, pp. 27-46.

KITTAY, E.F., *Love's Labor: Essays on Women, Dependency and Equality*, New York, Routledge, 1999.

KORSGAARD, C., 'Kant's Analysis of Obligation' in P. GUYER (ed.), *Kant's Groundwork of the Metaphysics of Morals: Critical Essays*, Lanham, Lowman & Littlefield, 1998, pp. 62-63.

KULTGEN, J., 'Consent and the Justification of Paternalism' in *The Southern Journal of Philosophy* 30(1992)3, pp. 89-113.

LEE, S., 'On the Justification of Paternalism' in *Social Theory and Practice* 7(1981)2, pp. 193-203.

LOEWY, E.H., 'In Defense of Paternalism' in *Theoretical Medicine and Bioethics* 26(2005), pp. 445-468.

MAY, L., 'Paternalism and Self-Interest' in *Journal of Value Inquiry* 14(1980), pp. 195-216.

MEULENBERGS, T. & P. SCHOTSMANS, 'The Sanctity of Autonomy?' in P. SCHOTSMANS & T. MEULENBERGS (eds.), *Euthanasia and Palliative Care in the Low Countries*, Leuven, Peeters, 2005, pp. 121-146.

MILL, J.S., *On Liberty*, ed. M. WARNOCK, Malden, MA, Blackwell Publishing, 2003.

NYS, T., 'The Tacit Concept of Competence in J.S. Mill's On Liberty' in *South African Journal of Philosophy* 25(2006)4, pp. 305-328.

O'NEILL, O., *Bounds of Justice*, Cambridge, Cambridge University Press, 2000.

O'NEILL, O., *Autonomy and Trust in Bioethics*, Cambridge, Cambridge University Press, 2002.

PULLMAN, D., 'Dying with Dignity and the Death of Dignity' in *Health Law Journal* 4(1996), pp. 197-219.

RILEY, J., 'J.S. Mill's Doctrine of Free Expression' in *Utilitas* 17(2005)2, pp. 147-179.

TAUBER, A.I., 'Historical and Philosophical Reflections on Patient Autonomy' in *Health Care Analysis* 9(2001), pp. 299-319.

TAYLOR, J.S., 'Autonomy and Informed Consent: A Much Misunderstood Relationship' in *Journal of Value Inquiry* 38(2004), pp. 383-391.

VERNON, R., 'John Stuart Mill and Pornography: Beyond the Harm Principle' in *Ethics* 106(1996)3, pp. 621-632.

WALDRON, J., 'Moral Autonomy and Personal Autonomy' in J. CHRISTMAN & J. ANDERSON (eds.), *Autonomy and the Challenges to Liberalism*, Cambridge, Cambridge University Press, 2005, pp. 307-329.

WERTHEIMER, A., 'Victimless Crimes' in *Ethics* 87(1977)4, pp. 302-318.

WOLPE, P.R., 'The Triumph of Autonomy in American Bioethics' in R. DEVRIES & J. SUBEDI (eds.), *Bioethics and Society: Constructing the Ethical Enterprise*, New Jersey, Prentice Hall, pp. 38-59.

1. BEYOND AUTONOMY AND PATERNALISM:
The Caring Transparent Self

Eva F. Kittay

"Caring seems to be the great motivator."
David W. Shoemaker[1]

"To say we should respect a right of autonomy is not to say
that we should ignore everything else."
Thomas E. Hill[2]

"Competence is a necessary but not sufficient condition...It
must be shaped at every step by the purposes of the healing
acts—by the good of the person who is ill—his bodily good,
of course, but also his concept of health, his value system,
and his sense of the kind and quality of life he thinks
worthwhile."
Edmund D. Pellegrino[3]

Autonomy has become the focal point for many who hold to a prin-
cipled approach to biomedical ethics, a development that has called
forth much critical attention. In this paper I will note but will not
dwell, as many already have, on the problem of elevating autonomy
to the central ethical precept of medical care. I also will not quarrel
with the position that paternalism is on the whole something to be
avoided, nor with the view that autonomy is on the whole a good
thing. Instead I want to call into question the dichotomy that is set up
between autonomy and paternalism in discussions of medical ethics.
That is, I question whether medical healthcare and practitioners must

---

[1] D.W. SHOEMAKER, 'Caring, Identification, and Agency' in *Ethics* 114(2003), pp. 88-
118.
[2] T.E. HILL, 'The Importance of Autonomy' in D.T. MEYERS & E. F. KITTAY, *Women
and Moral Theory*, Totowa, Roman and Littlefield, 1987, pp. 129-138.
[3] E.D. PELLEGRINO, 'Being Ill and Being Healed: Some Reflections on the Grounding of Medical Morality' in V. KESTENBAUM (ed.), *The Humanity of the Ill: Phenomenological Perspectives*, Knoxville, The University of Tennessee Press, 1982, pp. 157-166.

choose either to respect an individual's autonomy or to treat their patient paternalistically.

I will argue that there is a more satisfactory way of thinking about the obligations of medical personnel than these two options, one in which we recognise the dependencies and interdependencies that are inherent in the practice of medicine and health care and see medicine as a practice that must be at once a form of care and an exercise of expert knowledge[4] that fosters a shared understanding of an agent's neutral good, namely human health and human functioning. This alternative also acknowledges the limitations placed on medicine and healthcare because medical practice is itself situated in a larger context, one in which caring and the good of medicine and healthcare must compete with other goods and other conceptions of the good.

The first part of this paper will ask what is problematic in posing autonomy and paternalism as the dichotomous concepts guiding medical/health care. The problems that I identify are first, that the dichotomy encourages us to think of a sharp distinction between persons who are competent to make decisions on their own and those who are not; and second, it lessens the likelihood that we identify the role played by political, social and institutional contexts in constraining the self-understanding and decision-making of patients,

---

[4] We might add that "a tension which should be resolved in accordance with the principle of beneficence." Beneficence is sometimes equated with caring, and some who wish to counter the primacy of autonomy counter with the importance of beneficence. (See for example: A.V. CAMPBELL, 'Dependency: The Foundational Value in Medical Ethics' in K.W.M. FULFORD, G. GILLETT & J.M. SOSKICE (eds.), *Medicine and Moral Reasoning*, New York, Cambridge University Press, 1994, pp. 184-192; V.M. WOODWARD, 'Caring, Patient Autonomy and the Stigma of Paternalism' in *Journal of Advanced Nursing* 28(1998)5, pp. 1046-1052.) The position that Woodward takes and the data she presents to support a view is very close to my own. I believe the notion of a transparent self that I introduce below is what is required to deal with the cluster of issues she raises. But in this paper, I bracket the question of the relationship between caring and beneficence. I do so because when beneficence and care are used interchangeably, it is rarely clear what either term means. Insofar as beneficence is understood, as George Agich suggests it should be, "to be predicated not on the individual's isolated and abstract good, but on who the individual is in his concrete individuality," it comes increasing close to the conception of care that is put forward here. See: G.J. AGICH, 'Ethical Problems in Caring for Demented Patients' in S. GOVONI, C.L. BOLIS & M. TRABUCCHI, *Dementias: Biological Bases and Clinical Approach to Treatment*, Milano, Springer-Verlag Italia, 1999, pp. 297-308, p. 306. The discussion of care in this paper is meant to present a theoretical specification of care that may serve the principle of beneficence, but is not necessarily identical to it.

medical personnel and families around issues of health. An additional problem, which I point to is that when autonomy is operationalised as informed consent, we have a very narrow understanding of what it means to respect a patient's agency, one too narrow to do the work it is meant to do. The concerns I identify are, I believe, worries for both those normally thought to be competent and those usually classified as incompetent.

The second part of the paper will elaborate upon the alternative I propose. I argue that as the physician is both a carer and a skilled practitioner of medical science, the authority of the physician qua physician extends to her expertise, not to her role as a carer. As an expert practitioner she appropriately exercises her authority over the patient, based on her specialised knowledge and rightfully imposes on the patient that which is required by a conception of a certain good, the good of health. Carers, in contrast must be capable of setting aside their own concerns and preferences, sometimes even defer their own needs and preoccupations to be attentive to what the cared for requires in his dependency on the carer. As a carer, the physician (or other health care worker) has the responsibility not to interpose her own desires, values and conception of the good. Instead she must elicit the patient's own understanding of what the patient really needs, in light of what the patient, as *this* concrete individual, really cares about. Where the doctor cannot make herself transparent in the requisite way, she has a responsibility to be attentive to those who are or have been the true carers of the patient, that is those who are in a position to garner what the patient really needs in light of what that patient really cares about. At times the two roles are in conflict and call for different responses, but the physician must use her expertise in the service of her role as carer.

Seeing patients as having needs and dependencies defeats many assumptions of the autonomy of patients, but still leaves them with agency and individual concrete identities that demands the respect of the carer as she attends to patients' needs. Seeing patients in this way bridges the hard and fast divide of the competent and incompetent patient in the autonomy-paternalism model. Seeing both patient and doctor as enmeshed in relations of dependence and interdependence brings to the fore the institutional constraints on both the patient's autonomy and the ability of physicians to perform their dual capacity of medical expert and provider of care.

1. Autonomy

1.1 From Paternalistic Medicine to Autonomy

Within a liberal society, the assumption that persons are autonomous or competent to make important decisions for themselves, while defensible, is only questioned when evidence to the contrary appears. Concomitantly, the view that persons who are competent should be able to make decisions for themselves (and take responsibility for making those decisions) is equally an assumption questioned only in case an otherwise competent person is not in a position to make a rationally warranted decision.

Until relatively recently, the medical field has been exempted from these assumptions about persons because of the seemingly irremediable asymmetry of knowledge and skill between patient and medical caregiver. Instead the medical profession relied on a paternalistic model of care. The default assumption in the ethics, if not always the practice, of medicine and health care has given way to the value of respecting the autonomy of a person. The asymmetry once thought to be an obstacle to the autonomous decision making of the patient has become instead the basis for the requirement that the patient be provided with information adequate to making an informed decision, thereby acknowledging the importance of respecting the patient's autonomy even in the medical context.

Having experienced first-hand some of the well-intentioned but destructive consequences of paternalistic medicine, I concur with those who take this turn to patient autonomy as a good to celebrate. How far and fast we have moved from a time when paternalistic medicine, not patient autonomy, was the default is evident if we recall that as late as the 1970s in the United States it was considered good practice to treat patients as passive, as persons to be spoken about, not to. It was not long ago when doctors presumed that the truth (particularly when the news was bad) was to be confided in hushed tones to the nearest relative, not imparted to the patient herself; when doctors would not think of burdening patients with the details of the treatments they were to undergo or even the names of the medications they were prescribing.[5] Alan Buchanan reporting on

---

[5] It is difficult today to believe a practice I recall well from my youth: that in the United States, prescription medical containers had directions for use on the label, but not the actual names of the medicines. Physicians presumed that patients did not

a study of internists, surgeons, and generalists conducted in 1967[6] cited the conclusion that "there is a strong and general tendency to withhold from the patient the information that he has cancer. Almost 70 percent of the total group surveyed reported that their usual policy was not to tell the patient that he has cancer." Oken, whom Buchanan cites, also noted that "No one reported a policy of informing every patient."[7] We should not want to go back to those bad old days.

1.2 What is Autonomy?

What is autonomy and why do we value it? On a Kantian model, autonomy is the capacity to direct our actions by reference to the categorical imperative and take responsibility for those choices; on a model derived from John Stuart Mill, it is the capacity to direct the course of our lives; on a Rawlsian model it is the capacity to formulate and revise one's own conception of the good. Many contemporary authors characterise autonomy as a self-reflective capacity that permits an individual to be self-determining, to make choices for which one can take responsibility and choices with which one identifies, that is, an expression of who one is and what one authentically desires. On all these conceptions, the value of autonomy is seen to be a feature of persons (or on the Kantian model, of the will[8]) that both reflects and confers dignity on persons.

Some views such as the Kantian are contentful, a choice to act according to a maxim that we could not but will to become a universal law. Other views are purely procedural and require only a self-

---

need to know the name of the medication. I distinctly recall asking my physician the name of a medicine that he had prescribed and him saying to me: "What do you need to know the name of the medicine for?" All I needed to know was that he wanted me to take this medication and how he wanted me to take it. That names of medications have to be clearly indicated on the label is a relatively recent innovation. I believe, but have not been able to verify, that it was not until the passage of the Hazardous Labeling Act, passed in the 1960s, that all prescription medicines were labelled with the actual name of the medication.

[6] D. OKEN, 'What to Tell Cancer Patients: A Study of Medical Attitude' in S. GOROVITZ et al. (eds.), Moral Problems in Medicine, Englewood Cliffs, NJ, Prentice-Hall, p. 112, cited in A. BUCHANAN, 'Medical Paternalism' in Philosophy and Public Affairs 7(1978)4, pp. 370-390.

[7] Ibid. p. 372.

[8] See, for example: O. O'NEILL, Autonomy and Trust in Bioethics, Cambridge, Cambridge University Press, 2002.

reflexivity that identifies a desire as a desire I desire to have. Other procedural views may additionally invoke a set of competences, a "repertoire of coordinated skills that makes self-discovery, self-definition and self-direction possible."[9] Although the notion of autonomy has historically been tied to a conception of the self as an inner citadel, as the reverse of the heteronomy that directs us to act as social forces dictate, some who argue that the self is unavoidably and constitutively social nonetheless want to make room for autonomous judgments and actions. A relational understanding of the self argues that the development of autonomy in an individual, itself emerges from social interactions that provide us with competencies we need for autonomy. In turn, to be autonomous we respond to others' intentions and actions in social contexts that have determined and defined realms of legitimate autonomous action. These set the parameters by which we, for example, identify the difference between an autonomous act and a merely wanton act.[10]

Autonomy is a demanding capacity in the competences and cognitive capabilities it must engage. Just how demanding is evident in Gerald Dworkin's definition: "Autonomy is a second-order capacity to reflect critically upon one's first-order preferences and desires, and the ability either to identify with these or to change them in light of higher order preferences and values. By exercising such a capacity we define our nature, give meaning and coherence to our lives and take responsibility for the kind of person we are."[11] This is a tall order, especially when we are feeling ill, are facing overwhelming and confusing medical options, or are anticipating frightening medical outcomes. The demanding capacities required for autonomy may be beyond us when in our older years we experience diminishment or impairment of the sensory and cognitive capacities required to take in and process information.

Even a simpler, terser definition such as Sarah Buss's: "To be autonomous is to be a law to oneself; autonomous agents are self-gov-

---

[9] See: D.T. MEYERS, *Self, Society, and Personal Choice*, New York, Columbia University Press, 1989. See also: D.T. MEYERS, *Gender in the Mirror: Cultural Imagery and Women's Agency*, New York, Oxford University Press, 2002, pp. 20-21.

[10] For another view of the difference between an autonomous and a wanton act see H.G. FRANKFURT, *The Importance of What We Care About*, New York, Cambridge University Press, 1988.

[11] G. DWORKIN, *The Theory and Practice of Autonomy*, Cambridge, Cambridge University Press, 1988.

erning agents"[12] requires more than most of us can muster at the best of times. To be self-governing, a law to oneself, one must be capable of high cognitive functioning: one must understand the concept of law, know how to apply it to one's own actions, and be able to engage in self-scrutiny. In light of such demanding definitions of autonomy, it seems odd that autonomy has come to command centre stage in biomedical ethics, that is, in an ethics developed for a context where individuals are especially vulnerable and unusually dependent on others for the care and expertise that can determine their continued existence and well-being.

1.3 Autonomy Operationalised as Informed Consent

The philosophical concept of autonomy gets attenuated in the medical context and is largely operationalised as "informed consent." It is formalised in the requirement that the person receiving medical treatment has to sign an informed consent form. Informed consent surely has an important role in medicine: in medical research, for instance, it is indispensable. Moreover, given the need to externalise the intentional aspects of both autonomy and the respect for that autonomy, informed consent rightfully has an important place in good medical care.[13] Furthermore, it is understandable that providing information required to be certain that a patient's consent is informed, as well as obtaining that consent, have evolved into formal procedures, if only because the institutional structures within which medicine is practiced need to standardise the meaning and the enforceability of respect for autonomy.

1.4 Problems with Autonomy as Informed Consent

However, the ritualised and routinised consent (as patients in the US regularly experience it) in practice is often obtained by having a consent form shoved across the deck to a patient by an administrator

---

[12] S. Buss, 'Personal Autonomy' in *The Stanford Encyclopedia of Philosophy* (2002) on http://plato.stanford.edu/archives/win2002/entries/personal-autonomy.

[13] The idea of consent to medical treatment is often traced to the Nazi experimentation on human subjects. We can be quite certain that few if any would have consented to the experimentation that was enacted on their suffering bodies. Yet as such treatment was rarely justified as being for the benefit of the patients, malevolence, not paternalism would be the appropriate contrast to autonomy in these cases.

who waits impatiently for the patient's signature; or a form may be handed to a patient with a perfunctory explanation as the individual is about to go in for a major procedure. So while obtaining a patient's informed consent is required because it is a primary means by which to ensure that a patient's autonomy is respected, that consent is generally only a pale shadow of the autonomy that it is meant to embody.

Just as we can fault the process of obtaining informed consent from the patient's perspective, we can question the procedure from the care practitioners' point of view. For respect for autonomy requires honouring the consent obtained from the patient, even where there is no way to ascertain whether the consent was adequately informed or whether the patient was fully able to comprehend the import of giving such consent. Furthermore, the putatively autonomous decisions of the patient must be respected by the practitioner even when these decisions fail to accord with the care provider's own judgment of what would be best for the patient.

Respect for the patient's autonomy, adumbrated as it may be in the consent form and in the limitations institutional contexts impose, presumes a patient otherwise capable of autonomy in the fuller sense. Thus the model of respect for autonomy in medicine, especially something as operationalised as informed consent, does not pertain in all cases. It fails to encompass patients whose mental capacity is insufficient to understand the proffered information; patients who lack the judgment to make rational decisions; patients who cannot communicate their preferences in ways that are recognisable to medical personnel because they lack the capacity to express their preferences (through communicative impairments or cultural and language barriers). The model also does not cover situations that are likely to arise in long-term care or in the auxiliary care for acute conditions (that is, the nursing and daily care of patients). While we may be able to respect a patient's autonomy with respect to whether or not she is willing to go to a nursing home, a choice which can be made on the model of informed consent, it does little to address the nature of the living arrangements, the possibility of moving about freely in and out of the facility, nor the fine points of daily living.

These considerations reveal that in any particular situation the default assumption that we should accord respect to an individual's autonomy by assuring ourselves that the person in question is giving us her "informed consent" presupposes that we have already determined at least four questions:

1. Who can or cannot give informed consent? That is whether or not *this* is a patient capable of comprehending the necessary information in this situation.
2. Whether or not that consent can be obtainable from *this* individual in the prescribed fashion, namely through a formal mechanism, normally the signed informed consent form?
3. Whether or not this is a situation in which the caregivers can provide sufficient information and whether *this* situation is one for which consent is needed and if needed, lends itself to established formal means of consent.
4. If the options presented are real and realistic, so that if consent is given, it is reasonable that it be respected?

Doubtless the above does not exhaust the predeterminations that have been made when one asks for informed consent or when one acts in the absence of informed consent, nor is it the case that informed consent exhausts the means by which respect for autonomy is realised in the context of healthcare.

What is clear from this discussion however, is that this mode of operationalising autonomy fails many individuals who ought to have their desires and wishes recognised, even if they are not capable of the full blown philosophical conception of autonomy, or even if they are, but lack some communicative skills that can bring to bear their full capacities in the context of formalised procedures of consent. What also emerges is that there are many factors, besides the competence of the patient, that limit the possibility of respecting a person's autonomy. For example, policies that determine when and where consent is required; judgments on the part of medical administrators and health policy makers that determine whether a situation is significant enough (significant to whom? in whose view?) to warrant formal (or even informal) means of obtaining consent and determinations on the part of hospitals, medical insurers, physicians, etc. about what constitutes realistic opportunities for offering options, given economic, social and medical factors.

Furthermore when autonomy is conceptualised as formal consent, we may fail to see that autonomy can be violated in those situations where consent cannot be formalised or that demands made of patients and actions done to (or not done to) patients in these contexts have any bearing on autonomy. Clearly there are many policies in which a patient's consent is not and ought not to be sought. Whether patients ought to wear surgical gowns or their own clothing when wheeled into the operating room is not a matter for which a patient's consent is solicited, and if a patient were to question the policy, the staff may provide more or less satisfying reasons for the policy. This policy appears to have little bearing on the more important ways in which patients' autonomy should be respected. On the other hand, a policy subscribed to by most hospitals until relatively recently, that parental time with a young patient be limited to certain visiting hours, may well infringe on a parents autonomy rights with respect to their children.[14] When such policies were in place, there was no form for a parent to sign when he or she checked their child into a hospital to consent to leaving the child in the care of the hospital staff once visiting hours were over. It simply was not seen as a matter requiring informed consent, although many a parent had trepidations about leaving their sick children in the hands of strangers without their own parental oversight. Similarly there are the myriad of decisions made on the part of frail older people or older people with dementia without ever eliciting their or their family's consent. In fact formal consent forms for each of these matters would be utterly unmanageable and bizarre (and might do little to improve the patients' situation if the alternatives to signing the consent forms are still more unpalatable than the conditions they already endure). Yet these persons retain a measure of agency, and it accords

---

[14] "Forty years ago, it was common for a child's stay in hospital to extend for periods of weeks to months, and for them to see their parents infrequently during this time[…]. Parents were generally viewed as unwelcome visitors who upset their child and disrupted the hospital routine." AUSTRALIAN ASSOCIATION FOR THE WELFARE OF CHILD HEALTH (AWCH) 'AWCH 2005 National Survey Report — Sections 3, 4 and 5: Accommodation Facilities for Families, Childcare and Visiting Hours' (2005). Retrieved on March 6th, 2006, from http://www.awch.org.au/2005_AWCH_National _Survey_Report.htm. The same was true in the United States. Even today some hospitals have restricted policies, so that a children's hospital such as C. S. Mott's Children's Hospital (affiliated with the University of Michigan's Health Care System) includes as a response to the Frequently Asked Question "Can parents stay overnight with their kids?" the following statement: "Most Mott patient care units permit one parent or guardian to room-in overnight with the patient as the "parent partner in care." *However, this may not be available in all units,* so speak with your health care team once you arrive and read our *Staying Overnight Guidelines* for more information." (my emphasis, EFK). Even today it is not a given that you will be permitted to stay with your child. See: 'Frequently Asked Questions, C. S. Mott Children's Hospital' (2006), http://www.med.umich.edu/mott/pvguide/faq.html#overnight.

with their dignity to allow them agency insofar as they can appropriately exercise it. When their consent or choices are not sought or respected, they lose the precious dignity they ought to be able to retain.

As George Agich and others have remarked, the hallmark of autonomous decision making in the medical situation is generally taken to be the "big" decisions, whether or not to have surgery, or chemotherapy; whether or not to subject oneself to one medical procedure or another.[15] The smaller the treatment decision the more perfunctory the process of eliciting consent. Yet the larger, more medically complex and more urgent the medical need for a given treatment is, the less attractive the alternatives to a physician's suggested treatment are, and so ironically, the more irrelevant the required informed consent becomes. For example, a patient suffering from acute shortness of breath and experiencing significant chest pain may be urged to have an angiogram on the possibility that the symptoms are cause by a blockage in the left ventricle. As the patient arrives at the surgical appointment he is handed a consent form. The patient rightly wonders what purchase this consent form has, what relevance it has other than protecting the physician against a future law suit, as the patient has little choice but to rely on a physician's judgment in a matter such as this, since not doing the invasive diagnostic procedure could miss indications of a potentially fatal heart ailment.

In attempting to articulate the general presumption of autonomy and the predeterminations that go into operationalising autonomy as informed consent, we face the dichotomy between paternalism and autonomy. For we have to ask, if formalised mechanisms of informed consent seem not to be applicable to all patients and all medical or healthcare situations, are those individuals and situations always legitimately subject to paternalistic medical care? Is paternalism the

---

[15] Among George Agich's many writings on the topic, see: G..J. AGICH, 'Reassessing Autonomy in Long-Term Care' in *Hastings Center Report* 20(1990)6, pp. 12-17; G.J. AGICH, 'Actual Autonomy and Long-Term Care Decision Making' in L.B. McCULLOUGH & N.L. WILSON (EDS.) *Ethical and Conceptual Dimensions of Long-Term Care Decision Making*, Baltimore, John Hopkins University Press, 1995, pp. 113-136; G.J. AGICH, 'Respecting the Autonomy of Elders in Nursing Homes' in J.F. MONAGLE & D.C. THOMASMA, *Health Care Ethics: Critical Issues for the 21st Century*, Gaithersburg, Aspen Publishers, 1998, pp. 200-211; G.J. AGICH, 'Ethical Problems in Caring for Demented Patients,' 1999; G.J. AGICH, 'Seeking the Everyday Meaning of Autonomy' in *Philosophy, Psychiatry & Psychology* 11(2005)4, pp. 296-298.

only appropriate alternative to respecting patient autonomy, especially autonomy in the guise of informed consent?

2. Paternalism as the Contrary of Respect for Autonomy

Gerald Dworkin, in his latest conceptual analysis of paternalism, writes: "The analysis of paternalism involves at least the following elements...[1] some kind of limitation on the freedom or autonomy of some agent... [2] for a particular class of reasons." He acknowledges that "the exact boundaries of the concept is a contested issue."[16] Seana Shiffrin elaborates as follows: that A acts paternalistically toward B (through omission or commission) when A "aims to have an effect on B or her sphere of legitimate agency" by substituting A's judgment or agency for that of B's "directed at B's own interests or matters that legitimately lie within B's control" and that the substitution is undertaken on the grounds that A regards her judgment or agency to be superior than B's with respect to those interests.[17] The "limitation of freedom or autonomy" of which Dworkin speaks as is specified by Shiffrin in an attempt by A to affect B's interests or the sphere in which B legitimately exercises her autonomy or agency. The second conceptual element of which Dworkin speaks, "for a particular class of reasons," Shiffrin specifies as the intent on the part of A to affect B's interests and to substitute her judgment for B's *because* she believes her own judgment or agency to be superior with regard to affecting those interests.

I am generally persuaded by Shiffrin, whose account is among the most thorough available. There is a controversial part of her definition, namely the extension of paternalism to actions that are intended to affect not only B's *own* interests, but also those within a sphere that is within B's legitimate agency or autonomy. This means that A can act paternalistically toward B even when A acts not directly on B, so that if A (a ranger on a dangerous ski slope) prevents B (an aspiring skier) from skiing on the slope not because she is concerned for B's sake that he may injure himself, but is concerned for the sake of B's

---

[16] G. DWORKIN, 'Paternalism' in *The Stanford Encyclopedia of Philosophy* (2002) on http://plato.stanford.edu/archives/win2002/entries/paternalism.

[17] S.V. SHIFFRIN, 'Paternalism, Unconscionability Doctrine, and Accomodation' in *Philosophy and Public Affairs* 29(2000)3, pp. 205-250.

family's who depend on him (assuming here that the family falls within the sphere in which B legitimately exercises his autonomy or agency) and A does so because A thinks that her substituted judgment is superior to that of B.

As controversial as this position may be, it is also an appealing aspect of the definition, as it acknowledges that one's legitimate sphere of agency sometimes does include the interests of someone other than oneself. In other words, it acknowledges an important *relational* feature of autonomy. We can see how this operates when one considers the role of family members in the medical decisions of a relative. While a child, if young enough, may not be thought to have legitimate autonomy over her own health care decisions, the parent is generally thought to have such legitimate agency or control over the care of the child. Therefore when, for example, medical personnel are not sufficiently forthcoming about the foreseeable outcome of a child's medical treatment, even though we cannot say that their actions toward the child are paternalistic (as the child lacks a legitimate sphere of agency in this case), it may well be paternalistic toward the parents. This relational feature of our lives, which becomes more prominent when we are dependent through illness, disability, frailty or immaturity, is too often ignored in discussions of medical ethics. This point will be also be useful later when we consider surrogate forms of consent.

2.1 What is Wrong with Paternalism?

Is paternalism necessarily undesirable, so that to say that an action is paternalistic is already to condemn it? That is, is it tautological that paternalism is wrong and unjustifiable except as a lesser of two wrongs? Both Dworkin and Shiffrin attempt to be relatively neutral in their definitions of paternalism and aim for descriptive rather than normatively laden definitions. Dworkin's use of "interference" nonetheless has a normative flavour.[18] Shiffrin uses a neutral term, "substitution", but when she speaks of the "substitution" taking place within the realm of another's legitimate authority, agency, autonomy or control, this "substitution" sounds suspiciously like "usurpation."

---

[18] See: G. DWORKIN, *The Theory and Practice of Autonomy*, 1988. See also: G. DWORKIN, 'Paternalism' 2002.

Paternalism infringes on important liberties or on the special liberty that is autonomy and this, *prima facie*, is the first wrong of paternalism.[19] If paternalism is a wrong, it would seem to be so because it is an infringement on the liberty of another that is not justifiable in the terms that other such infringements are. It is, for instance, justifiable to limit one person's liberty because the said liberty interferes with the other's legitimate exercise of liberty. Paternalism, instead, is an infringement of a liberty in a sphere where the person interfered with has legitimate authority to exercise his or her agency. At least on utilitarian grounds it may be justifiable to interfere with such a legitimate exercise of agency (or liberty) if doing so will serve the greater good. But the good that is claimed to be served in cases of paternalism are goods that are generally within the sphere of the individual's legitimate authority, and so utilitarian grounds would not suffice to provide a justification for the paternalistic interference.

When another or a greater liberty or good is at stake which lies within the person's legitimate sphere of authority, interference may nonetheless be justifiable. For example, it is generally held to be justifiable to protect an individual's autonomy against a present choice that will rob the person of autonomy in the future. It is not clear whether we can count such interference as paternalistic, since the interference is justified on the grounds of protecting the other's *autonomy*. It is also arguable that a choice or action that precludes the possibility of any other autonomous action is itself not a product of autonomous reflection.

Interference in another's liberty may also be justifiable when the individual fails to understand that a greater liberty or good will be precluded by the present choice. Here again, it is not clear that the interference is not a case of paternalistic interference with another's autonomy, since autonomy requires adequate knowledge and understanding of the consequences of one's actions.

When paternalism is viewed as an interference in autonomy, many dispute whether any interference is justified as long as a patient is fully informed and competent to understand the consequences and impact of her decision. Paternalistic justifications in the case of medicine generally turn on some notion that to concede to a patient's wishes will produce great harm to that individual. Thus paternalism is justified on the basis of the principle that we should prevent harm.

---

[19] G. DWORKIN, *The Theory and Practice of Autonomy*, 1988.

Alan Buchanan argues that recourse to the "prevention of harm" principle is not well-grounded since appeal to the prevention of harm principle fails unless medical caregivers also ask what harm will result as an effect of the paternalistic interference.[20] However those who argue for the need for paternalistic interference rarely weigh the dodgy question of whether the harm that will occur from paternalist interference itself will be *greater* than the harm resulting from refraining from paternalistic interference.[21] Furthermore, he points out, in cases where the patient is incapable of understanding the situation or the available choices are generally ones where other caregivers or family members are involved. Justifying paternalism in these cases becomes justifying the paternalism towards the family or caregivers. But as in the previous situation, the prevention of harm justifications are not well-grounded, as the harm of not telling or deceiving or manipulating the family is rarely weighed against the anticipated harm of providing full information and allowing the family to choose.[22]

The harm done in the case of paternalistic interference includes the possibility of deceit and manipulating information, thereby undermining trust, even when the deceptions are justified for the patient's benefit. Making medical and other institutions trustworthy is critical if medical practitioners are to garner a justified trust. So in addition to failing to give due respect to the individual's autonomy, paternalism in medicine also undermines a relationship between medical practitioner and patient (and often the patient's family) based on trust.

Because if the very characterisation of paternalism already foretells the sorts of wrongs that paternalism engenders, it is difficult to say whether paternalism can ever be justified (except as a lesser of two evils). It appears that when the person who is treated paternalisti-

---

[20] A. BUCHANAN, 'Medical Paternalism' 1978.

[21] Buchanan argues that to justify paternalistic withholding of information by claiming that full disclosure will do patients great harm: "At least one other premise is needed: (2') giving information X will do greater harm to the patient on balance than withholding the information will." He adds: "The addition of (2') is no quibble. Once (2') is made explicit we begin to see the tremendous weight which this paternalist argument places on the physician's powers of judgment. He must not only determine that giving the information will do harm or even that it will do great harm. He must also make a complex comparative judgment." In: A. BUCHANAN, 'Medical Paternalism' 1978, p. 377.

[22] If the patient's well-being is within the legitimate sphere of authority or autonomy of the family, then there arises the additional question of why a physician should have the authority to interfere with the family, as the family is not the physician's patient.

cally is capable of autonomy, it is hard to find any truly justifiable
case of paternalism. Where the person treated in a putatively paternalistic fashion is incapable of autonomy, it does not seem appropriate to speak of the actions as paternalistic since then the sphere in
which the interventions occurred are not within the legitimate sphere
of that individual's autonomous actions, as that individual has no
such sphere, having no capacity for autonomy. Therefore it appears
that it cannot be correct to say that while paternalism is not justifiable
in cases where a person is capable of autonomy it is justifiable when
the person is incompetent. But it is only in these latter cases that the
case for the justifiability of paternalism appears to have any force.

This last conundrum suggests that perhaps the dichotomy between
paternalism and autonomy is not well-drawn and may not be as
helpful as it is thought to be.[23]

3. Problems with the Distinction Between Paternalism and Autonomy?

Several authors have suggested that the distinction, as it is usually
drawn, is not what is most interesting or important in thinking about
how a physician or other health care worker ought to treat a patient.
Our exploration of autonomy and paternalism has suggested at least
two reasons why the dichotomy between autonomy and paternalism
is ill-drawn and problematic. The first is that it draws a sharp line
between those competent to make decisions and those who are not.
This is a central problem addressed by both O'Neill[24] and Agich.[25]
The second problem is that the dichotomy ignores the role played by
the institutions of medicine and healthcare and larger social policy in
presuming and determining that certain arenas are legitimate spheres
of agency, autonomy and authority for competent and incompetent
agents. Here Shiffrin's analysis of paternalism will be helpful. Let us
consider each of these problems in turn.

[23] For various difficulties with arguments that autonomy is the reason that paternalism is objectionable, see: D. HUSAK, 'Paternalism and Autonomy' in *Philosophy and
Public Affairs* 10(1981)1, pp. 27-46.

[24] O. O'NEILL, 'Paternalism and Partial Autonomy' in *Journal of Medical Ethics*
10(1984), pp. 173-184.

[25] See note 15 above.

3.1 The Sharp Distinction Between the Competent and Incompetent

The sharp distinction between the competent and incompetent is of concern for both groups. Those who argue against the permissibility of infringing on autonomy must argue that in the case of persons generally judged competent, there is at least as much autonomy that remains as is needed to give informed consent, and that this is so in most cases. Yet an otherwise competent person who becomes a patient, whose judgment or other capacities are diminished by virtue of health, is effectively *abandoned* to make critical decisions on her own, and left to shoulder the responsibility of a decision she is ill-equipped to make.[26] The recognition that in these conditions we are at best only "partially autonomous," (in Onora O'Neill's phrase) is critical if we are to get proper care.

For those who are clearly incompetent — whose capacity for autonomy is clearly impaired, for example, those too young to be considered competent, individuals with severe mental retardation, the frail elderly with differing degrees of dementia, and those in a coma, a vegetative state or only partial consciousness — appear to be left without any voice in their medical fate. Although they may have no autonomy to undermine, important aspects of their agency and liberty can be sacrificed by the actions of a physician or other medical personnel who may feel justified in running roughshod over any such signs of agency. If we adopt the notion of partial autonomy, then we can countenance the possibility that in each case there are some pockets of agency (or in the case of those who have had but lost the capacity for autonomy, a history of agency) that still require consideration, voice and respect.

However we must note that if we accept the idea of partial autonomy, for both groups the question remains, what part is autonomous and what part is not? The notion of partial autonomy, while useful, still holds on to the competent-incompetent distinction, bringing the dichotomy within the breast or mind of a single individual.

---

[26] Woodward remarks that "In cases where the choice will clearly adversely affect the patient, Pellegrino counsels that practitioners need not be so neutral that they cannot indicate what they consider to be the best choice and proposes that no effort at persuasion is tantamount to abandonment." In: V.M. Woodward, 'Caring, Patient Autonomy and the Stigma of Paternalism' 1998, p. 1048. See: PELLEGRINO, E.D., 'Being Ill and Being Healed: Some Reflections on the Grounding of Medical Morality' in V. KESTENBAUM (ed.), *The Humanity of the Ill: Phenomenological Perspectives*, Knoxville, The University of Tennessee Press, 1982, pp. 157-166.

A still prior question may be posed by the standard treatment of autonomy and paternalism. Namely the question of what class of persons are we to include among "the clearly incompetent," even if we accept that "the competent" are, in conditions of illness, generally only "partially autonomous." Dan Wikler argues that to assume that the mildly retarded are incompetent by virtue of their diminished intellectual capacities, and therefore appropriate objects of paternalistic concern, asks the question of why we do not say that the normal are appropriate subjects of paternalistic concern for the intellectually gifted.[27] He argues that we deny the mildly mentally retarded the rights of self-determination about many (if not most) central life concerns because our understanding of these concerns derives from social institutions created by people with normal intelligence. We have the choice to continue to deny the mildly mentally retarded these rights or to alter the social arrangements so as to enable them to exercise far more self-determination. So we need to ask if it is morally permissible to deny these folks self-determination in central aspects of life simply because we choose to maintain institutions as we have fixed them rather than alter them or make suitable accommodations for those of different levels of intelligence?

Another challenge to the standard view of who should be counted among the incompetent is made by those who argue that we underestimate the capability of children. Priscilla Alderson has argued that we need to listen to children in making medical decisions that concern them, even such critical decisions as whether to undergo surgeries for achondroplasia.[28]

As these challenges suggest, it is not by all means clear that we can decide what groups are competent or not, much less if a particular individual is competent or not, or when the justifications for drawing such conclusions have a sound moral basis.

Another way to formulate the question is to borrow Shiffrin's notion of persons having a legitimate sphere of agency, and ask what persons have their (sphere of) agency legitimated? How high should the bar be set for an individual before her agency is accorded that legitimacy? Once again, the dichotomy between the competent and the incompetent, those who should be accorded autonomy and those

---

[27] D. WIKLER, 'Paternalism and the Mildly Retarded' in *Philosophy and Public Affairs* 8(1979)4, pp. 377-392.

[28] P. ALDERSON, *Listening to Children: Children, Ethics and Social Research*, London, Barnardos, 1995.

who should be treated paternalistically, risks running roughshod over whatever agency the "incompetent" possess. That is, we are likely to fail in giving neither the voices of the "incompetents", nor their relations to the persons they depend on, the respect they are due.

An alternative approach to the traditional paternalism/autonomy dichotomy that revisits the question of competency is suggested by Agich.[29] While O'Neill worries about the usefulness of the competent/incompetent divide because it "abandons" the competent to their putative autonomy, Agich is more concerned about the ways in which the "incompetent" lose voice in their treatment. George Agich, writing primarily about persons in long-term care, urges us to consider what it is that we most value in our ideal of personal autonomy and posits a conception of *actual* autonomy which is rooted in our identity and individuality that is still realisable by persons who are as dependent and cognitively impaired as frail elderly or demented elderly persons.[30]

Although an identity and individuality is still realisable by those whose are deeply dependent and cognitively limited, determining this requires caring persons who are willing and capable of being attentive to that identity and individuality. As Buchanan pointed out, we can reasonably suppose that when we speak of individuals too incompetent to make medical judgments on their own behalf, there is someone who has some responsibility for this person's well-being. What is the appropriate attitude towards those who have assumed such responsibility, that is, the family and other caregivers? How is their knowledge and concern for the ones they care for to be received by those who have the power and authority in the world of medicine and healthcare? There are two sorts of considerations that come into play. One has to do with those who may have no agency as yet (the very young infant) or no agency left (the vegetative patient). The other is of caregivers to people who clearly have some degree of agency, but who have limited or impaired judgment and have limited communication skills that caregivers need to interpret for them. Too often the families and caregivers, in both sorts of situations, are included under the paternalistic mantel.

Consider those who have not yet developed any agency, neonates, and the treatment of their families. In the past in the United States

---

[29] See note 15 above
[30] G.J. AGICH, 'Actual Autonomy and Long-Term Care Decision Making' 1995.

(and often still today), when a severely impaired neonate was born, it would be whisked away from the parents and sent to institutions forever out of sight of the unfortunate parents. Then and today, parents are asked to sign permissions for surgeries they can scarcely comprehend, given the stress and confusion of the moment. Usually, the parents of a child born with ambiguous genitalia are asked to make agonising decisions about genital surgery, often shortly after the birth. When the genital surgeries are not to treat life-threatening conditions or important functional limitations that require immediate attention, physicians are effectively framing decisions about sexual identity and normalcy as medical decisions, thereby compromising the parents' ability to form autonomous decisions about matters that they are no less informed about than physicians. The parents' dependence on the physician's judgment makes them susceptible to embracing the comforting mantel of paternalism.[31]

In treating an individual who is genuinely incapable of understanding the medical consequences of available options, yet who has the identity and individualism that Agich urges us to protect, the relationship between the medical personnel, the patient and the one(s) who care for the individual is a subject of controversy. Two possible routes are open. Beauchamps and Childress say in the fifth Edition of the Principles that it is the physician's obligation to act with beneficence (and nonmaleficence) towards the incompetent, and that there is no direct obligation to respect the judgment of the caregiver. However, some court judgments argue for the concept of "substituted judgment" (which Beauchamp and Childress oppose), where it is the judgment of a caregiver who may substitute her judgment for that of the patient, that has authority.

The notion of "substituted judgment" was established in the Supreme Court Case Superintendent of Belchertown State School v. Jos. Saikowitz in which the Court decided that incompetent persons must be accorded the "same panoply of rights and choices" as competent persons because they have "the same dignity and worth." If they are incapable of making a choice or give consent, a surrogate is to be appointed by the court who can render a "substituted judgment," either judging as that person would have us judge or judging

---

[31] See: E.K. FEDER, 'Doctor's Orders: Parents and Intersexed Children' in E.F. KITTAY & E.K. FEDER, *The Subject of Care: Feminist Perspectives on Dependency*, Lanham, Rowman and Littlefield, 2002, pp. 294-320.

so as to concord with that person's best interest. Whether a surrogate can make these judgments, whether one applies a best interest standard, and who, if anyone, is to make a substituted judgment are highly contested issues.

One objection to substituted judgment is that it makes little sense to determine what a person judged incompetent would have desired. Consider those who previously were competent and while competent voiced a choice. The incompetent person she has become may have very different interests and concerns from those of the previously competent self. In the case of someone who never has been thought competent, the question becomes: How or on what basis does one determine what such persons would want were they competent? Were they competent, could they even be thought to be the same person?

Whether the individual in question had or had not been previously competent, the possibility of abuse looms large in the case of surrogate judgments. Furthermore, there are times, such as in the infamous case of Terry Schiavo, when it is difficult to determine who should serve as surrogate. In the Schiavo case two sets of parties each claimed to be the only one to truly care about Terry Schiavo's well-being, her parents and her husband, and while her parents insisted on keeping her alive although she had been declared to be in a vegetative state for years, her husband argued that she would never have wanted to be kept alive in that condition.[32] How is one to decide whose judgment is the correct substituted judgment or who best represents the interests of the incompetent person?

Yet even in light of these difficulties, the concept of substituted judgment may still be important to affirm. Without a surrogate who knows and speaks for the individual, that individual may be denied the liberty to refuse treatment the medical establishment may feel obligated to provide; treatment that it may only withhold when the patient herself refuses the treatment. Few reject the notion that we have the right to make autonomous judgments about whether to

[32] For a brief narrative of the Terry Schiavo affair, see: 'Terri Schiavo' in Wikipedia (2006) on http://en.wikipedia.org/wiki/Terri_Schiavo.

[33] Superintendent of Belchertown State School V. Jos. Saikowitz in *MA 370 N.E Reptr*, MASS Supreme Court, 2d(1977), p. 417. For a broader discussion of legal autonomy based rights and profoundly mentally disabled persons see N.L. CANTOR, 'The Relation between Autonomy-Based Rights and Profoundly Mentally Disabled Persons' in *Annals of Health Law* 13(2004) pp. 37-80.

accept or refuse treatment. If no provision is made for a surrogate to provide a "substituted judgment," the denial of a fundamental liberty is inevitable. It is considerations such as this that lead to the "substituted judgment doctrine" in Belchertown v. Saikowitz. [33]

In Belchertown v. Saikowitz the court determined who was to be the surrogate making the substituted judgment. I would maintain that only someone well acquainted with the person, her values, desires etc., is situated to provide a substituted judgment and then, only if that person cares about the well-being of the incapable person for that person's own sake. It is such a one that ought to make the medical decisions and give informed consent as he or she, I believe, is the one most capable of reflecting the individual's agency and the individuality and identity that Agich argues we rightly value in the notion of autonomy. The absence of such an individual in the life of a truly incompetent person is itself a sign of a deep injustice that has been done to the person.

The dichotomy between respect for autonomy and paternalism sets the default assumption at autonomy, an assumption that is not pertinent to those judged incompetent and often not applicable in the medical context for those judged competent. In this section, I have argued that this default renders the identification and legitimisation of whatever agency is available to "incompetent patients" problematic; and it risks giving insufficient attention to the needs of the "competent patient" in times of stress and in the face of the expertise possessed by the medical personnel.

3.2 The Autonomy/Paternalism Dichotomy and the Social Context of Medical Decision Making

Now let me turn to the second set of difficulties surrounding the autonomy/paternalism dichotomy. These concern the diversion of attention away from the social, political and institutional settings in which decisions are being made, when the focus is on autonomy and paternalism. The point is perhaps best made through a set of examples.

Example 1

This case involves the consent for the experimentation on prospective inmates of Willowbrook, a state institution for retarded persons that became the symbol of all that was wrong with institutionalising persons with cognitive disabilities. In the proposed experiment, child inmates were to be injected with a hepatitis virus in a trial test for a hepatitis vaccine (hepatitis was rampant at Willowbrook, because many patients were incontinent and the virus spreads through faecal matter). The idea of the study was justified by its proponents because first of all hepatitis in children is milder than in adults; secondly, because the children would be brought to a well-equipped, well-staffed hospital where they would not be subject to many of the other diseases also prevalent at Willowbrook; thirdly, because the test subjects could possibly acquire a mild immunity to the disease after exposure; and finally, because only children who had parents and who would be asked to consent would be subject to the experiment. Opponents to the proposal objected to experimentation on a population that could neither give consent, nor object to their parents granting permission, and they questioned whether such consent on the part of the parents could really be free and well-informed. Opponents also pointed out that there were alternate ways to control hepatitis (such as through gamma globulin injections) and that the experimenting with a vaccine was not the only way to get desired results. Yet what remained unquestioned when the focus was on whether the children and their parents were being treated paternalistically or having their autonomy respected, were the conditions at Willowbrook giving rise to the certain spread of hepatitis. These included overcrowding, understaffing, inadequate hygiene — in short, the moral scandal that was Willowbrook. Posing the question of whether the experiment was justified on the grounds of autonomy or an instance of justified paternalism entirely misses the most crucial moral question, which was why such institutions were allowed to exist at all.[34]

Example 2

This example underscores the role of socio-economic class as framing questions of paternalism and autonomy. A New York Times article examining medical services in New York City featured three individuals of different socio-economic classes all of whom suffered

---

[34] This case appears in T.L. BEAUCHAMP & J.F. CHILDRESS, *Principles of Biomedical Ethics*, New York, Oxford University Press, 2001.

from heart disease.[35] The article details the immediate care each
received, the period following the immediate treatment, including
their diet and the support each received from family, friends and
physicians and the outcome in each case. The treatment, follow-up
and outcome varied considerably by socio-economic class, as is
illustrated by the choice of hospital in the three cases. The upper
middle class executive suffered a heart attack in a midtown Man-
hattan street while accompanied by business colleagues who immediately called for an ambulance. He was given the choice of
whether to go to a nearby private teaching hospital, or a still nearer
public hospital. The executive chose the private hospital, where he
was met by his doctor, received excellent care, and was out of the
hospital and back on his feet within weeks. The middle class
African American office worker was asked if he wanted to go to a
far away private hospital or a nearby and more affordable public
institution. He "chose" the latter, although it was hardly a choice
since the superior hospital was a significant distant away from
where he lived and the additional medical bills would have been
prohibitive. The third person was a poor white woman who
worked as a cleaning lady and lived in one of the boroughs of New
York. She was not feeling well while at home and resisted calling
for an ambulance since she was not covered by insurance. When
her husband finally called, she was immediately taken directly to a
nearby public institution; she was never given any choice at all.
Here all three individuals were "competent" but their ability to
exercise judgment about their treatment was severely curtailed by
their ability to pay, by where in the city they were, and by their
friends' or associates' ability to aid them.

Example 3

Here I would like to call attention to the fact that medical personnel
(in the United States at least) have time pressures and unrealistic
work schedules that derive from a number of factors including the
way medical services are financed. Attempting to provide truly adequate information to their patients is a struggle, especially where the
patient requires special attention. Just as providing nursing that

---

[35] J. SCOTT, 'Life at the Top in America Isn't Just Better, It's Longer' in *The New York Times*, May 16, 2005.

recognises autonomy within the routinisation of care under such conditions becomes problematic. Nor can they deal with patients in a sufficiently leisurely manner to assure themselves that their patients truly understand what was said to them or what the autonomous wishes of their patients are. Respecting autonomy is only given lip-service and doctors and other personnel act in accordance with expediency and some form of triage.[36]

Example 4

The last example speaks to the cultural blindspots and misunderstandings that make a mockery of the idea of informed consent and that dissolve all expectations that patients can act autonomously. Ann Fadiman's essay *The Spirit Catches You and You Fall Down* describes the disastrous case of two caring attentive Hmong parents, a young child suffering from severe seizure disorders and well-intentioned physicians who were as clueless about the Hmong understanding of seizures as the parents were of Western medicine.[37] The parents, while concerned, repeatedly refused to follow the directives of the physicians. The parents were not compliant because they were unfamiliar with certain aspects of Western medicine and did not share the view that seizures were an unalloyed evil. In particular, they did not fully understand the instructions; they were not looking for a complete cessation of seizures but only for a lessening of the worst of the effects; they viewed medicine as only required for treating the symptoms as they occurred; they were inadequately apprised of side effects of the medications: and they saw no reason to subject their child to the side-effects of the medications when the child stopped having seizures, as they were unfamiliar with the idea that seizure control required a maintenance dose of the medication. The physicians lacked the understanding that might have allowed them to interact with the parents in an effective manner and so they reluctantly went so far as to forcibly

---

[36] For some empirical data gleaned from nurses that supports the contentions above, see Woodward, who writes: "Routine and overload risks both good care and the ability to facilitate patient autonomy" in V.M. WOODWARD, 'Caring, Patient Autonomy and the Stigma of Paternalism', p. 1048.

[37] A. FADIMAN, *The Spirit Catches You and You Fall Down*, New York, Farrar, Strauss, and Giroux, 1997.

separate the child from the parents, with disastrous consequences. The child, who received excellent and loving care at home, languished, suffered increasing irreversible brain injury, and nearly died in the care of well-meaning strangers.

From the perspective of the parents, the physicians were clearly infringing on their legitimate sphere of authority even when they were insistent on having the child on a maintenance regimen of pills that lessened the alertness of their child. Yet the physicians were insisting on standard, well-documented treatment for the control of severe seizure disorder. From the perspective of the physicians, to grant autonomy to parents who refused to be compliant with the medical directives to keep the child on anti-seizure medication would have been to jeopardise the well-being of the child. Yet their decidedly paternalistic intervention to remove the child from the home of the noncompliant parents had catastrophic results, at least as bad as if the parents were granted their legitimate authority with respect to the child's well-being. These parents were people capable of acting autonomously and for the child's best interests, but in circumstances which failed to provide an adequate translation across cultures, were incapable of acting as the physicians expected autonomous and competent parents to act. Instead they were treated as incompetents and the physicians were forced into the position of acting paternalistically, with terrible results for the child as well as the parents.

In the first example, the proposed Willowbrook hepatitis vaccine trials, the debate concerning autonomy and consent diverted attention from the social injustice and evil that made Willowbrook possible. The second example concerns the institutional constraints that make a mockery of the "fully informed" part of the consent, the stand-in for the principle of autonomy in medical procedures. The third example directs attention to the way socio-economic factors are determinants in respecting the autonomy of patients. The last example dwells on one such determination, cultural difference, especially as it plays out in the case of parents and their child.

Each example points to the need to move beyond the discourse of autonomy and paternalism if we are to recognise how factors outside the physician patient relationship impact on the meaningfulness of the respect for autonomy and constrain the possibilities of preserving the agency of patients regardless of their degree of competence.

4. The Caring Transparent Self and Limitations of Medical Authority

4.1 An Ethic of Care and the Transparent Self

An ethic of care elaborates on the idea of a relational self. At the heart of the idea of a relational self is the idea that we are dependent beings. As there is no time that we are more dependent than when we encounter the need for health and medical care, if we are to find a more satisfactory conception of the relation between medical personnel and those receiving care we must begin by recognising our inherent vulnerability and dependency. The relationship in which we receive the care that sustains us through these periods of inevitable dependency helps to constitute who and what we are.

The positive valence of notions such as independence, self-sufficiency and autonomy, prevalent in the Western, modern worldview (and especially virulent in the US) is accompanied by the idea that dependency is always to be avoided. Yet should dependency be viewed in so negative a light?

Alastair Campbell speaks of the need not only to respect autonomy, but also to respect dependency, that is, the need for it and the inevitable fact of it, the persons on whom we depend when ill and who depend on us when we are well.[38] Dependency, he maintains is "the foundational value in medical ethics," and cites a passage from Oliver Sacks:

> "Though as a sick patient in hospital, one was reduced to moral infancy, this was not a malicious degradation, but a biological and spiritual need of the hurt creature. One had to go back, one had to regress, for one might indeed be as helpless as a child, whether one liked it, or willed it, or not. In hospital one became again a child with parents (parents who might be good or bad), and this might be felt as 'infantilizing' and degrading, or as a sweet and sorely needed nourishing."[39]

While Campbell sees dependency as a positive good, I think we ought to see it as a neutral but inevitable aspect of human existence. Perhaps a better response than Campbell's positive assessment of dependency per se, is Alasdair McIntyre's positive view of what he calls the virtues

---

[38] A. CAMPBELL, 'Dependency: The Foundational Value in Medical Ethics' 1994.
[39] Oliver Sacks cited in *Ibid*.

of *acknowledging* our dependency.[40] McIntyre's argument that there are virtues in acknowledging our dependency does not limit these virtues to the medical context. These virtues, he claims, need to pervade our life. When we try to deny or take flight from our own inevitable human dependency, we come to stigmatise those who cannot be independent once they have passed childhood: the ill, those with many sorts of disabilities and frail elderly persons. Even children are not given their full due, a regard for their agency and due consideration of their judgment because of the low esteem in which we hold being in a state of dependence. The stigma of dependence makes us despise being ill still more than the pain, discomfort and threat of death that illness brings in its wake. We reject and isolate those who are dependent on others for basic tasks because of physical or mental impairments. Although self-determination is a strong human value, insisting on it at the cost of masking dependencies makes self-esteem that is tied to self-determination terribly precarious; and the state of independence much in need of defending. Because dependency is devalued, the work of caring for dependents is devalued. Because we want to deny our dependency when we need it most, we make those who provide that care invisible.[41]

Most pertinent to our considerations here is that we tend to view care as a subsidiary of medicine and healthcare rather than the overarching concept. The *care* in medical care is seen as secondary, and the task associated with caring is assigned to subordinates, in part at least, because it does not comport with the elevated stature of the medical profession and our flight from and stigmatisation of dependency. To remove these blinders, we need to acknowledge the inevitable dependency in human life and the work of medical care to attend to us in our dependency.

If medical care is a species of care, then it is a practice to which an ethic of care is pertinent. An ethic of care articulates the moral

---

[40] A. MacIntyre, *Dependent Rational Animals: Why Human Beings Need the Virtues*, Peru, Open Court Publishing, 1999.

[41] Thus we justify the poor wages and working conditions of dependency workers and enshrine the racial and social hierarchies that determine who does the work of care. I have argued elsewhere that a society, indeed a world, (since care has global dimensions) that is truly just demands a society that acknowledges dependency and the importance of care. See: E.F. Kittay, B. Jennings & A. Wasunna, 'Dependency, Difference and the Global Ethic of Longterm Care' in *The Journal of Political Philosophy*, 13(2005)4, pp. 443–469.

demands of caring relations. It is also an orientation toward the ethical that has at times been contrasted with a justice orientation. When we take justice as the central moral orientation, autonomy as self-governance or self-determination emerges as a predominant moral theme. Associations between persons are to respect the autonomy of each agent so that relationships of autonomous agents emerge from voluntary agreements that are acceptable to each party. On the societal level, voluntary contractual relationships between autonomous persons result in arrangements which allow each party the maximum liberty consistent with an equal liberty for the other party or parties. This picture of the autonomy of all parties is necessary to get a liberal theory of justice off the ground.

Within an ethic of care, the self is not the autonomous subject of liberal theory, but always a self-in-relationship, enmeshed in a web of relationships. Within an ethic of care, what is required is respecting the relationships which constitute the self and within which the self is entwined. An ethic of care requires respect for the integrity of the self, but the self as it is supported and maintained through relationships.

On the assumption that equal and autonomous selves engage in social cooperation, their relationships are conceived of as voluntary and mutually advantageous to each party (why would equal autonomous selves agree to any other terms of cooperation?). Interactions between parties in situations of care are not necessarily interactions between equals and are not always voluntarily chosen: children do not chose their parents any more than parents chose their children; a patient showing up in an emergency room does not engage a physician out of choice but out of necessity and generally has little choice over who that physician should be. Nor are parents and children equals, as patients are not the equals of their skilled physicians and trained medical staff.

Is health care carework, or as I call such work when it deals with those who are inevitably dependent, "dependency work"? Is medical care dependency work? Much of what a nurse does is dependency work, but it is not entirely so. To the extent that that nursing has been professionalised, it becomes less so. Is a physician a dependency worker? To some extent she is. She provides care for people who are inevitably dependent; but professionalised work has few of the markers of dependency work. The other-directed and non-self-interested character of the work is surely similar to dependency work. The difference is seen in features of medical practice that are associated with status: the emphasis on its intellectual character, a training that draws on "generalized and systematic knowledge," the autonomy claimed for the professional through self-regulatory codes of ethics, and the existence of voluntary and autonomous organisations.

Furthermore, while dependency work involves concern for the general well-being of the dependent person, medical care is concerned with a person's well-being only as that well-being can be served by medical practices. Dependency work, in other words is *functionally diffuse*,[42] professionalised work is functionally specific. Yet what those medical personnel are largely engaged with are persons who are dependent and in need of care.

The relations of care as characterised by an ethic of care, while based on the practice of care, are not purely descriptive but have normative force. Care is a practice, but underlying the criteria of good care is an ethic of care. While some, perhaps many, care relationships are in fact paternalistic, the *ethic* of care speaks of what *good* care is, what in terms familiar to medicine, "best practice" demands. An ethic of care can be characterised by a set of virtues, foremost among these are attentiveness and responsiveness to another's needs and vulnerabilities. Such responsiveness requires a self that sees itself in a relationship with the other. It is a self that can attend to the other and make itself permeable to the needs of another through an empathetic identification with the other. In other writings I have spoken of such a self as a transparent self:[43] "The demands of dependency work favour a self accommodating to the wants of another; that is, a self that defers or brackets its own needs in order to provide for another's."[44]

---

[42] R.B. DARLING, 'Parent-Professional Interaction: The Roots of Misunderstanding' in M. SELIGMAN (ed.) *The Family with a Handicapped Child: Understanding and Treatment*, New York, Grune and Stratton, 1983, pp. 95-121.

[43] E.F. KITTAY, *Love's Labor: Essays on Women, Dependency and Equality*, New York, Routledge, 1999. E.F. KITTAY, 'When Care Is Just and Justice Is Caring: The Case of the Care for the Mentally Retarded' in *Public Culture*, 13(2001)3, Special Issue, The Critical Limits of Embodiment: Reflections on Disability Criticism, pp. 557-579.

[44] Capturing the sense of what I mean by "a transparent self" is a passage from Carl Elliot and Britt Elliot: "Clearly it is much easier for me to imagine what it would be like for *me* to undergo a given experience than it is for me to imagine what undergoing that experience is like for *another* person. That sort of imaginative leap would require me to imagine what it is like to share another's particular, subjective point of

As dependency work is an indispensable feature of any human society, it is crucial that some persons can muster the demands of being a transparent self. What are these demands? A transparent self does not allow its own needs or vision of the good to cloud its perception of another's needs, and so offers no resistance to its response to another (except, of course, when such a response would be in direct violation of a well considered and deeply held moral belief or conception of the good). The perception of and response to another's needs are neither blocked by nor refracted through our own needs and desires. A transparent self attempts to intuit and respond to the other's own sense or understanding of their own good, and does so for the other's *own* sake.

Of course, no self is ever truly transparent in this sense, but such transparency is a benchmark for the self-conception of the individual who cares for a dependent person. It is a regulatory ideal. One might say that it is an altruistic ideal. But while altruism is often seen as morally supererogatory, this ideal is *required* of dependency work, work which is itself a requirement of human life lived together with others. The transparency of this self is placed in stark contrast to the self of the liberal tradition of rights and utilities, wherein it might be viewed as a heteronymous rather than an autonomous self. This is not to say that altruism goes unrecognised in that tradition; it is acknowledged but it does present a problem. "The problem [...] is not how the interests of others can motivate us to some specific policy of altruistic conduct, but how they can motivate us at all" writes Thomas Nagel.[45]

What motivates the carer is that she cares about the other and that she cares about caring. As David Shoemaker, writing of care as an ethical concept says, "care is the great motivator."[46] It motivates us to perceive or understand ourselves to have certain needs and desires. It also motivates the one who cares either for or about another to care about the other's caring. Caring about the other means having a concern for what the other cares about insofar as the other cares about

---

view, to imagine what it is like to *be* another person — and this is another matter entirely." In: C. Elliot & B. Elliot, 'From the Patient's Point of View: Medical Ethics and the Moral Imagination' in *Journal of Medical Ethics* 17(1991), pp. 173-178, p. 173.

[45] T. NAGEL, *The Possibility of Altruism*, Oxford, Clarendon Press, 1970, p. 79.

[46] D.W. SHOEMAKER, 'Caring, Identification, and Agency' 2003, p. 91.

it; it means attending to what the other needs as the other comes to sense or understand a need.[47]

We have only hinted at what it is it that this transparent self must make herself transparent to. To the aches, pains, discomforts and basic needs of a dependent other? Most certainly. But these are immediate needs not life plans. How does one make oneself transparent to the life plan of another? Moreover have we here recreated the split between the competent and the incompetent? The competent have a life plan, they have an autonomous vision, in whose service the physician is asked to exert his efforts. The incompetent are left with moans and groans — basic needs that need to be inferred.

The putative competent and incompetents as divided for us by the autonomy/paternalism dichotomy however, each share something that the transparent self most needs to be responsive to. It is what the individual in question cares about. David Shoemaker has made the useful point, "If we attach free agency to willing action, then, and willing action consists in the action I genuinely want to do, and what I genuinely want to do depends on what I care most about in any particular situation, then free agency is grounded ultimately in care."[48] I remarked earlier that the transparent self cares about caring. Shoemaker notes that "Indeed, caring requires such emotional vulnerability." This insight into agency and care makes it easier to

---

[47] Of course, an ethic of care cannot require us to care about what the other cares about, when what the other cares about violates our own considered judgment of either how a moral person ought to act, or care about a good that is in stark opposition to the good as we understand it for ourselves. For instance, a caregiver to a wounded Nazi SS Commander may care about giving succour to a fellow human being without caring for the Nazi ideology adopted by the cared for. And if healing the Nazi only allows him to carry out murderous acts, the caregiver might consider if she has any obligation to provide such care. Similarly, a physician who is asked by a person with all her limbs intact to amputate one or more limbs because that person claims not to feel whole with such "extraneous" limbs, a physician who understands her duty as a physician to never cut off limbs except to save a life is under no obligation to oblige the owner of these limbs. Although an ethic of care recognises that not all actors in a moral situation are equal in the sense of being equally empowered or equally situated, it nonetheless acknowledges the moral parity of each actor. Thus each one is equal to another in terms of one's entitlement to care about different things and these entitlements would have to be such that one person's entitlement is not an infringement on that of another — in a manner analogous to the granting of the maximum number of liberties that are compatible with the maximum number of liberties of all others. That is, no one is entitled to care about murdering others, about destroying what others care about, etc.

[48] D.W. SHOEMAKER, 'Caring, Identification, and Agency' 2003, pp. 103-04.

appreciate how difficult it is for medical professionals to care, to make themselves vulnerable in this fashion, especially given the current construction of medical institutions.

Although I have tried to question the centrality of the idea of autonomy in medicine and health care, at this point in our investigation it is worthwhile to return to autonomy and consider what about the idea of autonomy makes it such an attractive concept in medical ethics. When we think of autonomy as the capacity and right to choose among possible options, we have to admit that we often want to make choices for ourselves. But is it not only the value of being able to choose that makes autonomy an attractive ideal? What we most want when we want autonomy is to preserve the capacity to act and care about that which we care about. Shoemaker makes a number of salient points with respect to the value of being able to care about that which we care about: "When I care about something, this caring produces a web of desires;"[49] "Losing one's capacity to care means losing one's identity as a coherent agent."[...] "Motivationally efficacious desires and judgments flowing from my cares, therefore, flow from me: they get any authority they have only derivatively, reflecting what I genuinely want — what I authorize on my behalf — only insofar as they depend on my cares, the set of emotional investments making me the agent I am."[50] This sort of agency is often associated with our cognitive capacities, but it is open not only to those who are competent to make medical choices but also to those who are incompetent, for they do not lose the capacity to care about what they care about when they lose the capacity to make rational judgments.

4.2 Distinguishing the Caring Self and Paternalism

Care relationships arise out of a need to be attended to, or to answer to the needs of the other. Where care is care of dependents, the carer may not be interacting with another self that can articulate its own needs and wants. When one is incapable of being articulate about one's needs we require the other to feel their way into our perspective, our need. Why do I say that these relationships are not, need not be, and should not be paternalistic? Are not care relationships paradigmatically paternalistic?

---

[49] *Ibid.* p. 95.
[50] *Ibid.* p. 114.

Care relationships have many characteristics that suggest paternalism. They are often relationships between unequals in which one person, A, is or at least appears to be, better equipped to access resources for and attend to the needs of another, B, than B himself is. If paternalistic relationships are ever acceptable, it is when they are between unequals, C and D, where C bears the relationship to D that A bears to B. When A cares for B, A acts to promote the welfare of B, for B's own sake.[51] In the case of paternalism, C similarly acts to promote D's welfare, although it is less clear if the second situation pertains. However, those who act paternalistically generally claim to be acting for the sake of the other, and not for their own good or some abstract good. Recall Shiffrin's definition of paternalism: A acts paternalistically toward B (through omission or commission) when A substitutes A's judgment or agency for that of B's "directed at B's own interests or matters that legitimately lie within B's control" because A believes her judgment to be superior to that of B's.

We have noted that on Shiffrin's definition and that of many others, it is questionable whether one can even speak of acting paternalistically toward someone who is, for example, too ill to care for himself even concerning matters that otherwise "legitimately lie within's B's control" since these matters may not lie within B's control when he is so ill that he loses the capacity to have control over that sphere. Nor is it clear through Shiffrin's analysis whether it even makes sense to say of a mother or father caring for an infant or young child that they act paternalistically, since so little is within the control of an infant or young child. Thus much of carework lies outside of the domain of actions that can rightfully be called paternalistic. The more difficult cases are those where B will retain some agency, but not in a position to be in full control, and A considers that her judgment is nonetheless superior to that of B even where B retains the capacity for some agency, because that judgment is compromised by B not having full agency. Consider for example, the parent of a child old enough to be in control of what he eats, who insists that his child eat what he the parent, says the child should eat because the parent believes that his opinion of what is good for the child is superior to that of the child. Or that of a physician who insists on her patient taking painkillers and overrides the patient's

---

[51] S. DARWALL, *Welfare and Rational Care*, Princeton, Princeton University Press, 2002.

objections that he doesn't like painkillers (because of their side-effect of drowsiness or their addictive properties, or because he associates taking painkillers with being weak) on the grounds that the patient is too distraught (or pigheaded or proud) to understand what is good for him. In these cases it is hard to determine if the behaviour of A (the parent or physician) is simply good caring without paternalism (because B, in this case, lacks the full control of that domain or sphere of activity that B might otherwise have) or if it is caring *with* paternalism where A substitutes her judgment for that of B's, and that does result in a better outcome (as judged by both A and B) for B.

There are cases of caring (or, at least what passes for caring) that are unquestionably paternalistic. A physician who is convinced that patients do less well when told the truth about a terminal disease and so keeps this knowledge from his patient may well claim that he deceives his patient with cheery news because he cares about the patient and believes that this is the right way to care for the patient. The action seems to be a paradigm of paternalism. If one believes that good caring is not paternalistic, then one would have to maintain that a physician is not practicing good care when she acts according to the maxim that one ought not to speak truthfully to a patient with a terminal disease. As I will point out below, there is a way in which an ethic of care would say just this, but there is another way in which it would not say that about some instances of this behaviour.

How then is care as an ethical ideal to be distinguished from a paternalistic care? A non-paternalistic carer is a carer whose self is transparent in the way discussed above. A non-paternalistic carer not only perceives another's need and attempts to act to alleviate that need, she also tries to intuit, or in some way understand, *how* the cared for needs to have the needs fulfilled. She attempts to understand the vulnerability of the cared for from the perspective of the one needing care and to do for that person what that person would want to do for himself; to act as an affordance to the other's needs. In many ways this is the antithesis of paternalistic behaviour.

The *pater* in paternalism is the figure of authority, the figure who has the power to impose his will on another and has the authority to do so, especially when it is purportedly for that individual's own good. He has that authority by virtue of the place he has in a recognised hierarchy purportedly constructed for the good of all within it. The authority of the transparent self derives from the authority of the

person for whom she cares, the authority vested in each of us to tend
to our needs and to that about which we truly care. When we do not
have the means by which to be active in meeting these concerns,
another must take over if we are to survive or thrive. When that
other is appropriately situated (in terms of proximity, the appropriate familial relationship, or personal relationship or skills) we effectively turn to the other as a proxy. Nevertheless, as an ethic of care
understands selves as always being in relation to others, we are
always in the process of acting as proxies for one another to some
extent and in various ways.

The picture of the world from which paternalism arises is quite different. Paternalism emerges as a virtue within hierarchical institutions, particularly within a patriarchy, where, it is true, relationality
rather than autonomy is viewed as essential to identity and virtue of
all (except perhaps the patriarch himself).[52] Yet *authority* over the
lives of others is vested in the patriarch. The good of the patriarch
and the good of the members of his dominion are one, and that one
good is the good as the patriarch sees it. This origin of paternalistic
authority is suspect not only where the guiding vision is that of
autonomy for all, where each person has a right to fashion her own
conception of the good; it is also suspect in an ethic of care, where the
carer is to give care that embraces the good of the cared for and
where the carer makes herself transparent to the other's good. Thus
an ethic of care, and with it the concept of the transparent self, are
notions that count neither autonomy nor paternalism as virtues. To
move beyond the dichotomy of autonomy and paternalism, we have
recourse to another mode of attending to one in need of medical
attention or seeking other healthcare, the mode of the caring transparent self.

Let us revisit some of the examples of where neither respecting
autonomy nor acting paternalistically seemed satisfactory. Consider
for example the case of the nursing home residents, who are fragile
and have dementia, and who have little say in what they are fed and
other aspects of their daily lives. These persons cannot be accorded a
strong sense of autonomy as they have a diminished sphere in which
they have legitimate agency. At best we can say that they are par-

---

[52] Aristotle's discussion of the family in the *Politics* is a paradigm of such a view.
The virtue of wives and slaves are defined in terms of their relationship to the patriarch.

tially autonomous in O'Neill's sense or that they need to be accorded "actual autonomy" in Agich's sense. But how are we to ascertain what part of a partial autonomy they should retain and how are we to accord these individuals the actual autonomy that respects their individuality and identity? Formal consent forms, even if signed by surrogates would only serve well in cases where there are defined procedures that could reasonably be consented to or refused. Neither the individuals we are dealing with, nor the situation that is of concern lend themselves to formalised procedures. What is required, I propose, is a staff that is trained and encouraged to serve as caregivers who can make themselves transparent to the individuals that they are caring for, and also a set of policies that would support caregiver's judgments when the judgments arise out of such a transparency of a caring self. Financial and other institutional supports are needed to support and encourage this sort of caregiving.

Consider once again the physician who lies to his patient about the patient's terminal condition. In many cases, such behaviour is simply paternalistic and unwarranted. But when a family comes to the physician and says that they have previously carefully discussed the question with the patient and that the patient has clearly said that she would not want to be told that her illness is diagnosed as terminal, then a physician who insists on "respecting the patient's autonomy" and bluntly tells the patient that she has 6 months to live is acting no more responsibly than the physician who always lies. Whether or not to tell a patient her fate, depends on the character and background of the patient. The physician must set aside any preconceived views of whether or not to tell, and must be guided by an understanding of the patient through attending *with care* to what it appears the patient wants. Even when the family has intervened to insist that the patient would not want to know, both family and physician have to be attentive to indications that the patient, who is now in the position of being a very ill person who may have sensed the truth of her condition, may have changed her mind and at this juncture wants to and needs to be told the truth. At times a physician may see such a change before the family does and must help the family to see that this is how their relative wants to be treated at this point. Acting according to maxims in such cases is not good caring, whether the maxim is to never deceive or to always deceive.

Once again however, the interaction between patient and physician is never merely an interaction between two individuals. Physicians need a certain training to act as transparent selves; they require the time to pay attention to the signs of how a patient wants and needs to be treated and cared for; they need institutions that will support judgments that derive from this sort of responsiveness to the patient. If a physician makes a determination (generally together with close family members) that this is one of those times when the patient really should not be told, they must not be undermined by a policy that insists that all patients *must* be told because only this respects the patient's autonomy. Time does not permit us to revisit all the sorts of encounters that we have touched upon, and these two may suffice to indicate what needs to be in place if we are to look beyond the dichotomy of autonomy and paternalism to a sounder view of the relationship between medical personnel and patients.

However this is not the end of the story, because the physician has an authority that derives neither from a patriarchal hierarchy nor from a willingness to attend to the needs of one who cannot care for herself.

4.3 Medical Expertise and Authority

Although medical care, and healthcare more broadly, should be understood as a species of care, clearly the highly technical and highly skilled nature of much healthcare makes medicine and healthcare also a branch of a technologically sophisticated practice and science. The authority with which medical judgments by medical personnel are vested derive from their training and accumulated expertise. Here it is helpful to introduce a distinction between an agent neutral good and an agent specific good. An agent specific good is a good that is endorsed as a good by a particular, or endorsed as a good for some particular agent, but not necessarily a good for all or a good all endorse. The study of philosophy is a good for some, for those who like and believe in the value of philosophy. It is not something most think should be foisted on all. Health however is generally viewed as an agent neutral good, it is a good we generally wish for ourselves and we believe that most would wish for themselves. This is not to say that each and every one of us would and should choose health over all other goods, agent-specific and agent neutral, as health is, after all, an instrumental good. It is a good we wish for ourselves so that we might have other goods, some intrinsic like happiness, some instrumental like being able to work. *All things considered* then, health is a good that would be endorsed by all as, at least, an instrumental good. Even if we count it as an intrinsic good, it is not the only intrinsic good nor the *summum bonum*. The science and the practice aimed at producing health and overall functioning then is an 'agent-neutral' good. Moreover that which medicine and healthcare aims at is the good not from the perspective of a particular doctor or patient but as an agent-neutral good of medicine. This medical good is an agent-neutral good because it depends neither on an individual physician's vision of a good more broadly conceived, nor on that of the patient or the patient's family or social context. Being free of cancer is not simply something that is good from any particular patient's point of view or any particular physician's point of view, it is a good as medicine as a body of knowledge and a practice goes. There also must be a shared understanding that this practice is indeed an agent-neutral good.

As a medical professional, the physician appropriately uses her authority to insist on certain courses of action for a patient (with whom he shares an understanding of the agent-neutral good of medicine), when that authority is grounded in an expertise based on an agent-neutral conception of a good, the good of a well (not diseased) functioning (not necessarily in a species typical way) body which can allow an individual to be an agent in the world who acts on what that individual really cares about. The physician interprets that good as it is appropriate to the condition of her patient.

That the agent neutral good of medicine must be a shared understanding will help us see why the tale that Ann Fadiman tells in *You Fall Down and the Spirits Catches You* went so badly. For the Hmong parents who sought medical attention for their child's seizures, such a shared understanding of a medical good was absent. Although the parents thought that health was a good, what the family and physicians did not share was the good of medicine as it pertained in the case of seizure activity. For the family medical intervention meant *alleviating* the condition, not ceasing *all* seizure behaviour, because for the Hmong seizures were not perceived as the unalloyed evil in the way that Western medicine views it. From the Hmong perspective, seizures are visits from the spirits and make the child a special medium of the spiritual world. At the same time, the parents understood that severe seizures could endanger their child, and it was only this aspect of seizure activity that they wanted to control.

Where there is a shared understanding of an agent neutral conception of a good, as understood by a particular science and practice, even such a deceptive practice as providing a placebo may not be an instance of paternalistic medicine, or at least no more paternalistic than forcibly preventing someone from crossing a bridge when he does not know of its immanent collapse. The latter scenario is a classic example of the infringement of a liberty for the good of the person whose liberty is curtailed that does not count as paternalistic, because were the person to know of the bridge's instability she would not have wanted to have crossed it. The forcible prevention of the act is justified both by the fact that the person acted upon was lacking some crucial information, that there was no possibility to impart the necessary information before the necessary intervention, and because both the person who prevented the other's bridge-crossing and the potential bridge-crosser shared an understanding of an agent-neutral good, namely not crossing a bridge when doing so would result in plunging into the sea. If one can argue that if the patient truly understood the consequences of her choice, she would not make that choice, but would choose the course of action dictated by the physician, then it seems we no more have a case of paternalism than we do in the bridge-crossing scenario.

Here the physician acts by way of his authority that derives from his expertise, and he must be clear that the actual expertise required in this particular instance warrants countering the patient's. As a carer, the physician needs to ascertain the source of the resistance (assuming circumstances permit it), or if there is a competing good to the agent neutral good they both endorse. I cited the good of being free of cancer as an agent neutral good of medicine. Even in such an obvious case, it is possible that a particular patient's understanding of the good may render such an agent neutral good less desirable than other agent-specific or agent neutral goods. Health as we noted earlier, is for most at least, only an instrumental good. An elderly person, for reasons that have to do with something that she cares about even more than she cares about her own life, at least at this advanced age, might prefer not to receive radioactive treatments or chemotherapy, even when these would be critical to saving her own life and no other means of achieving the same end are available. This person might have spent much of her life caring about and working for a safer, cleaner environment and might not want to be part of the radioactive or the chemical pollution to which such therapies can contribute. As she reckons it, unleashing such radioactive materials into the environment is, all told, a greater evil than the loss of her own life, at least at this time in her life.

While a physician is not one who ought to make such a reckoning (at least not without telling patients in advance that he is opposed to these treatments on non-medical grounds), a respectful and caring attitude of a physician may make her to acquiesce to such a judgment when it is a well considered judgment. To do otherwise is for the physician to use his medical authority to make judgments which go beyond the shared understanding of the agent-neutral good of medicine, but which may be overridden by another good that the patient cares still more deeply about than her own health. To understand and empathise with his patient, to act in the capacity of a carer, the physician must make himself transparent to the deeply held convictions of the patient, even as he advocates for the agent-neutral good of a medical procedure that would be likely to save the patient's life.

Note that the argument being employed here to accept the patient's desire not to undergo radiation treatment is not an argument about respecting the patient's autonomy, although such an action would do that. Instead it is an argument about what is demanded of a good medical caregiver, in particular a caregiver who attempts to ascertain how to assist and help the patient in ways that honour what the patient truly cares about, given a shared understanding of the good of medicine. A patient might insist on refusing radiation therapy because she fears the accompanying ailments that go with radiation therapy and her talk of polluting the earth just may be a subterfuge. A good carer, one who is trained to be attentive to the particularities of the cared for, will try to discern the underlying fear or the deep conviction and will be responsive to whichever factor is operative. The good medical carer will propound the shared understanding of the agent-neutral good of the prescribed medical treatment but will also recognise the equally important role of carer and the virtue of a carer's transparent self.

Medical personnel, however, cannot help but hold conceptions of the good that lie outside of the domain of medicine per se. Unfortunately, many situations that appear to call for medical intervention are highly influenced by more than the shared understanding of agent-neutral goods. Some of these situations are difficult to parse. Is intersexuality a medical emergency as doctors have so frequently told anxious parents, one requiring immediate surgery to normalise the genitals (aside from conditions such as hypospadias and congenital adrenal hyperplasia which are urgent medical conditions correctible without correcting the condition of intersexuality)? Or is it the judgment of the physician that genitals that look normal, even when functionality is compromised, are a necessity for each and every child? While the former draws upon the physician's medical expertise and a judgment based on the good of health, the latter calls upon a prevalent, but not necessarily an agent-neutral conception of the good, as many adults who have had the various surgeries needed to "correct" intersexuality have been arguing.[53] Is the judgment that dwarfism resulting from achondroplasia should be "treated" with limb lengthening a medical judgment drawn from an agent-neutral understanding of the good of medicine? Or is it a "surgical fix" for a condition that has no medical need for surgery but a need for greater awareness and accommodation by society at large? Is the decision to tell or not tell a patient that she has cancer something that relies on an agent-neutral medical good? Does the physician herself not want to face the terrible truth that her expertise cannot extend as far as a cure in this situation? Or are there good medical studies that indicate that patients do better when they are or are not told the truth? And does how well a patient does when given or not given the bad news, depend on the patient's own attitude to facing death?

Whenever the answer is "no" to the question of whether the decision is based on the agent-neutral good of medicine, or even, if the answer is "I'm not sure" the practitioner needs to avoid overstepping her medical authority. When a physician uses her authority as a medical expert to promote what is in fact not a shared understanding of an agent's good (and in particular, the physician's conception of what that good is as it pertains to the person in question) then the physician uses the authority as a *pater* in a patriarchal household would: to maintain that his version of the good is *the* version of the good, and to impose it whether or not others concur.

4.4 The Relational Autonomy of Both Patient and Practitioner

There are also times when physicians or other medical personnel find themselves promoting a treatment (or avoiding treatment) with the

---

[53] See: FEDER, E.K., 'Doctor's Orders: Parents and Intersexed Children' 2002. Also see http://www.isna.org/ for more information about the opposition to such surgeries by those who have undergone them.

authority of the medical expert, but which neither comports with the good as judged by them as medical experts, nor the agent-specific good that they themselves hold to, nor the good as the patient views it. It happens when medical agent-neutral good is trumped by expedience, by the (in)ability of the patient to pay or the (un)willingness of insurance companies to provide coverage, by exigencies that pertain to policies or demands by medically uninformed or indifferent social, economic or political institutions or by prejudices that go unnoticed by practitioners. These are exigencies that interfere with both good care and good medicine. The emphasis on medicine as a practice of care, and on medical and health personnel as caregivers, direct them not only to act with a transparency of self, but to attend to such circumstances that undermine the possibility of such care. Just as the possibility of autonomy for the patient is not merely a matter of the capacity for *autonomy* for an *individual*, the possibility of being a medical caregiver who meets the ideal of a transparent self with an authority that derives from a medical expertise is not merely a matter of an *autonomous individual* medical caregiver. We need to be aware of relevant dependencies and interdependencies, ones that are obscured in talk of autonomy and paternalism, but which have a place in an ethic of care. Among these are:

- The dependency of the patient on the doctor and other medical personnel who in turn is dependent on a specific sort of training, in which norms are transmitted along with specific skills.
- Economic dependencies that include that of the patient to others and others to the patient, dependencies which impact on the ability of patients to pay for medical costs on which the practitioners in turn depend and which determine the sort of care they are free to provide.
- The dependency of medical personnel on the institutions in which they operate both for resources and policies.
- The availability of the medicine dependent on public policy.
- The social dependencies of social connections and education that the patient and practitioner alike bring in to the healthcare situation.
- Cultural dependencies that help determine how the medical situation presents itself to the patient, and how the patient appears to medical personnel.

Many of the above were elaborated upon when we looked at the limits of discussions of autonomy and paternalism as well as when we looked at the obstacles to acting as a transparent self in the medical context. Many of these dependencies and interdependencies are implicated in the notion of a relational autonomy, where the self is viewed as situated in a matrix of relationships.[54] We can never truly choose just for ourselves because we never are only isolated individuals, and this is true of physician and patient alike. When we look at the broader social and political contexts in which we operate and which help determine the choices we make, our capacity to make choices and the parameters which set the choices before us, we politicise our understanding of a relational self.

5. A Final Word

Charles Fried notes that there are times when "the doctor must see himself, as the servant, not of life in the abstract, but of the life plans of his patients."[55] When the doctor sees himself as "the servant of the life plans" of his patient, he is taking on the role of a carer. Here the doctor is called on to be a carer in a sense that is more akin to the dependency worker, as his task is now not functionally specific but functionally diffuse. As "servant" suggests, this role does require the physician to assume a transparency of self. His role here is not to presume that his understanding of the good is the patient's good. That *is* paternalistic. His role is instead to intuit, either through extended discussions or through careful attentiveness to his patient's condition and to discover what this ailing and dependent individual requires in the form of care, whether it is medicine, consultation or even handholding.

What I have presented as the role of the medical caregiver may appear to be too demanding a role for medical personnel. A care ethic is in fact a very demanding ethic, one that can be personally costly as well. Furthermore as I have pointed out, institutional arrangements make it very difficult if not impossible for many in health care to carry out both roles of medical expert and carer. In addition there

---

[54] For a discussion of relational autonomy in bioethics see: A. DONCHIN, 'Understanding Autonomy Relationally: Toward a Reconfiguration of Bioethical Principles' in *Journal of Medicine and Philosophy* 26(2001)4, pp. 365-386.

[55] C. FRIED, *Medical Experimentation: Personal Integrity and Social Policy*, Amsterdam, North Holland Publishing, 1974, cited in G. Dworkin, *The Theory and Practice of Autonomy*, p. 113.

are cultural and social barriers to understanding that cannot easily be overcome in attempting to come to a shared understanding of goods or to come to see another's good as a good. The barriers may be such that only a deep and intimate connection makes it possible to establish the necessary communication and trust. For these and a host of other contingencies, the physician may not be able to play the role of the transparent self.

What is one to do when faced with these obstacles? First it is important that the doctor and other health care workers must understand their limitations and their own dependencies. Aside from institutional dependencies, in many cases a physician is dependent on those close to the patient to enable her to be an adequate caregiver. Where the patient is cognitively immature or impaired (infants, the mentally retarded, the Alzheimer's patient) it is often presumptuous for a physician to attempt to usurp the role of a transparent caring self.[56] For those who are inevitably dependent even outside the medical setting it is of critical importance to be connected to those who care for them and for professionals to respect that relationship of dependency. Such an individual's well-being is intertwined with the well-being of those on whom she depends. This sort of connection is not limited to persons who are dependent, although it is most evident in such cases. It is for them to offer judgments when there is a real choice in medical care. Such judgments, if made by a caregiver's transparent self, must respect and protect the agency of the dependent person. The agency of the less than fully competent may be attenuated, but it is never entirely absent. Even those in a vegetative state have a residue of agency which is preserved in the memory of those who care for them. The judgments of caregivers should have the status of "substituted judgment," legally and morally. Yet in spite of this a "substituted judgment" must not be a paternalistic judgment which is likely to override or ignore what remains of the other's agency. A "substituted judgment" needs to be one that issues from a transparent self who is attentive to the needs, desires and agency (however attenuated) of the person for whom they care.

A good doctor cares to the extent that he can make himself transparent to what the other cares about and makes medical choices

---

[56] The exception to this rule is cases where one sees evidence of neglect, abuse or mistreatment of the person who may be unable to speak for herself. Then the physician cannot trust the putative caregiver to act as a transparent self.

based both on his special expertise and his empathetic understanding of what is important and meaningful to the patient, that is, what the patient cares about caring about. Where the medical professional who attempts but meets the limitations of his own ability to be transparent, he engages those who can interpolate for him. In this way he respects each person's particular way of being in the world and carefully considers the limited authority his knowledge and position provides. To fulfil his role, he will have to depend on a set of well ordered institutions that support his practice of medical care and without which he is restricted in his ability to apply his expertise and provide medical *care*.

To capture these realities and necessities, do we really need the terms paternalism and autonomy? Do they obscure more than they illuminate?

References

AGICH, G.J., 'Reassessing Autonomy in Long-Term Care' in *Hastings Center Report* 20(1990)6, pp. 12-17.

AGICH, G.J., 'Actual Autonomy and Long-Term Care Decision Making' in L.B. McCULLOUGH & N.L. WILSON (eds.), *Ethical and Conceptual Dimensions of Long-Term Care Decision Making*, Baltimore, John Hopkins University Press, 1995, pp. 113-136.

AGICH, G.J., 'Respecting the Autonomy of Elders in Nursing Homes' in J.F. MONAGLE & D.C. THOMASMA (eds.), *Health Care Ethics: Critical Issues for the 21st Century*, Gaithersburg, Aspen Publishers, 1998, pp. 200-211.

AGICH, G.J., 'Ethical Problems in Caring for Demented Patients' in S. GOVONI, C.L. BOLIS & M. TRABUCCHI (eds.), *Dementias: Biological Bases and Clinical Approach to Treatment*, Milano, Springer-Verlag Italia, 1999, pp. 297-308.

AGICH, G.J., 'Seeking the Everyday Meaning of Autonomy' in *Philosophy, Psychiatry & Psychology* 11(2005)4, pp. 296-298.

ALDERSON, P., *Listening to Children: Children, Ethics and Social Research*, London, Barnardos, 1995.

AUSTRALIAN ASSOCIATION FOR THE WELFARE OF CHILD HEALTH (AWCH), 'AWCH 2005 National Survey Report — Sections 3, 4 and 5: Accommodation Facilities for Families, Childcare and Visiting Hours' (2005). Retrieved March 6th, 2006, from http://www.awch.org.au/2005_AWCH_National_Survey_Report.htm.

BEAUCHAMP, T.L. & CHILDRESS, J.F., *Principles of Biomedical Ethics*, New York, Oxford University Press, 2001.

BUCHANAN, A., 'Medical Paternalism' in *Philosophy and Public Affairs* 7(1978)4, pp. 370-390.

BUSS, S., 'Personal Autonomy' in *The Stanford Encyclopedia of Philosophy* (2002) Retrieved Winter 2002, from http://plato.stanford.edu/archives/win2002/entries/personal-autonomy

CAMPBELL, A.V., 'Dependency: The Foundational Value in Medical Ethics' in K.W.M. FULFORD, G. GILLETT & J.M. SOSKICE (eds.), *Medicine and Moral Reasoning*, New York, Cambridge University Press, 1994, pp. 184-192.

CANTOR, N.L. 'The Relation between Autonomy-Based Rights and Profoundly Mentally Disabled Persons' in *Annals of Health Law* 13(2004), pp. 37-80.

DARLING, R.B., 'Parent-Professional Interaction: The Roots of Misunderstanding' in M SELIGMAN, *The Family with a Handicapped Child: Understanding and Treatment*, New York, Grune and Stratton, 1983, pp. 95-121.

DARWALL, S., *Welfare and Rational Care*, Princeton, Princeton University Press, 2002.

DONCHIN, A., 'Understanding Autonomy Relationally: Toward a Reconfiguration of Bioethical Principles' in *Journal of Medicine and Philosophy* 26(2001)4, pp. 365-386.

DWORKIN, G., *The Theory and Practice of Autonomy*, Cambridge, Cambridge University Press, 1988.

DWORKIN, G., 'Paternalism' in *The Stanford Encyclopedia of Philosophy* (2002) Retrieved Winter 2002, from. http://plato.stanford.edu/archives/win2002/entries/paternalism

ELLIOT, C. & ELLIOT B., 'From the Patient's Point of View: Medical Ethics and the Moral Imagination' in *Journal of Medical Ethics* 17(1991), pp. 173-178.

FADIMAN, A., *The Spirit Catches You and You Fall Down*, New York, Farrar, Strauss, and Giroux, 1997.

FEDER, E.K., 'Doctor's Orders: Parents and Intersexed Children' in E.F. KITTAY & E.K. FEDER, *The Subject of Care: Feminist Perspectives on Dependency*, Lanham, Rowman and Littlefield, 2002, pp. 294-320.

FRANKFURT, H.G., *The Importance of What We Care About*, Cambridge, Cambridge University Press, 1988.

FRIED, C., *Medical Experimentation: Personal Integrity and Social Policy*, Amsterdam, North Holland Publishing, 1974.

HILL, T.E. 'The Importance of Autonomy' in D.T. MEYERS & E.F. KITTAY (eds.), *Women and Moral Theory*, Totowa, Roman and Littlefield, 1987, pp. 129-138.

HUSAK, D. 'Paternalism and Autonomy' in *Philosophy and Public Affairs* 10(1981)1, pp. 27-46.

KITTAY, E.F., *Love's Labor: Essays on Women, Dependency and Equality*, New York, Routledge, 1999.

KITTAY, E.F., 'When Care Is Just and Justice Is Caring: The Case of the Care for the Mentally Retarded' in *Public Culture* 13(2001)3, Special Issue, The Critical Limits of Embodiment: Reflections on Disability Criticism, pp. 557-579.

KITTAY, E.F., JENNINGS, B. & WASUNNA, A. 'Dependency, Difference and the Global Ethic of Longterm Care' in *The Journal of Political Philosophy* 13(2005)4, pp. 443–469.

MACINTYRE, A., *Dependent Rational Animals: Why Human Beings Need the Virtues*, Peru, Open Court Publishing, 1999.

MEYERS, D.T., *Self, Society, and Personal Choice*, New York, Columbia University Press, 1989.

MEYERS, D.T., *Gender in the Mirror: Cultural Imagery and Women's Agency*, New York, Oxford University Press, 2002.

NAGEL, T., *The Possibility of Altruism*, Oxford, Clarendon Press, 1970.

OKEN, D., 'What to Tell Cancer Patients: A Study of Medical Attitude' in S. GOROVITZ, R. MAKLIN, A. JAMETON, J. O'CONNOR & S. SHERMAN (eds.), *Moral Problems in Medicine*, Englewood Cliffs, NJ, Prentice-Hall, 1976.

O'NEILL, O., 'Paternalism and Partial Autonomy' in *Journal of Medical Ethics* 10(1984), pp. 173-184.

O'NEILL, O., *Autonomy and Trust in Bioethics*, Cambridge, Cambridge University Press, 2002.

PELLEGRINO, E.D., 'Being Ill and Being Healed: Some Reflections on the Grounding of Medical Morality' in V. KESTENBAUM (ed.), *The Humanity of the Ill: Phenomenological Perspectives*, Knoxville, The University of Tennessee Press, 1982, pp. 157-166.

SCOTT, J., 'Life at the Top in America Isn't Just Better, It's Longer' in *The New York Times*, May 16, 2005.

SHIFFRIN, S.V., 'Paternalism, Unconscionability Doctrine, and Accomodation' in *Philosophy and Public Affairs* 29(2000)3, pp. 205-250.

SHOEMAKER, D.W., 'Caring, Identification, and Agency' in *Ethics* 114 (2003), pp. 88-118.

Superintendent of Belchertown State School V. Jos. Saikowitz in *MA 370 N.E Reptr*, MASS Supreme Court, 2d(1977), p. 417.

'Terri Schiavo' in *Wikipedia* (2006). Retrieved from http://en.wikipedia. org/ wiki/Terri_Schiavo

WIKLER, D., 'Paternalism and the Mildly Retarded,' in *Philosophy and Public Affairs* 8(1979)4, pp. 377-392.

WOODWARD, V.M., 'Caring, Patient Autonomy and the Stigma of Paternalism' in *Journal of Advanced Nursing* 28(1998)5, pp. 1046-1052.

2. AUTONOMY AS A PROBLEM FOR CLINICAL ETHICS

George J. Agich

The problem of autonomy for clinical ethics is eminently practical; hence, considering autonomy in clinical contexts requires more than theoretical analysis or justification of concepts. This is not to say that these treatments of autonomy are irrelevant to clinical ethics, but rather that theoretical treatments of autonomy do not fully engage the full range of questions arising in the course of caring for patients. In this contribution, I focus not on the familiar acute care context, which has been subject of most bioethical attention, but the context of long-term care. I will argue that this context helps us to see why a phenomenologically-informed understanding of autonomy is essential for addressing everyday clinical ethical questions and concerns arising in the course of patient care.

I.

Several features of long-term care make it an important subject for examination of the meaning of actual autonomy. First, although autonomy has a wide and diverse range of meanings, virtually all commentators agree that the term etymologically involves self-governance, which is often taken to imply independence. Thus, long-term care presents a paradox, because it is characterized by significant types of dependence and incapacity. Individuals in long-term care do not always satisfy the basic conditions that are taken-for-granted in many discussions of autonomy. They are neither robustly functional nor independent.

Many individuals in long-term care are significantly dependent on their caregivers in ways that are quite uncommon for adults. Their functional incapacities compromise the expression of their autonomy in ways that complexly extend beyond simply altering their decisional capacity that is seen by many theoretical accounts as the main expression of autonomy. Because their personal care needs override other concerns and interests, loss and grief are dominant experiences associated with their adaptation to their needs for care. To be sure, situations of conflict that typically engender the appeal to autonomy and patient rights in the acute care also occur in long-term care, but they are not my primary target, primarily because they do not differ significantly from the conflicts arising in acute-care medicine and also because they occur only episodically within the course of everyday care.

Second, the ethical challenges in long-term care extend far beyond the dramatic conflicts that dominate mainstream bioethical attention. In comparison, the concerns in long-term care settings are far more mundane; they lack the drama of high technology acute care medicine. These concerns of long-term care might appear to be more psychological or psychosocial than ethical. Rather than conflicts involving decision making, long-term care involves concerns about the quality of care that might seem far more affective than cognitive in nature, so there might be doubt about the contribution that philosophical reflection can make in this setting.

Long-term care occurs in a wide variety of settings: in the home, chronic care institutions, or nursing homes rather than hospitals or clinics. Long-term care involves relationships that typically fall outside the paradigmatic professional relationships like physician-patient or nurse-patient relationships. For example, low-paid and often unskilled or custodial caregivers, family, or friends provide the majority of day-to-day care and supportive services for old people. Only episodically do a wide variety of health professionals get involved in the delivery of specialized services. Hence, the normative framework of professional medical or nursing ethics cannot be expected to clarify the day-to-day interactions that occur in long-term settings.

Third, except for the theoretical questions about the persistence of self or personhood when an individual undergoes changes associated with dementia, most of the attention to autonomy in long-term care involves the extension of ethical analyses worked out in acute care contexts, such as advance directives, informed consent (particularly, in preadmission agreements), surrogate decision-making, and patients' rights. Long-term care commonly involves other situations that are truly unlike those typically addressed in acute-care bioethics. These day-to-day services constitute an important reason to examine what autonomy might mean in the mundane circumstances of long-term care.

Individuals receive long-term care, because disability or incapacity creates a need for assistance with a broad range of everyday activities or specialized health care services. Although decisional crises and conflicts involving informed consent, decision-making capacity, and surrogate decision-making punctuate long-term care, these well-recognised topics of acute-care ethics are less prominent. Long-term care mainly involves everyday care giving interactions quite unlike the high technology-driven, life-and-death paradigms that have received the most bioethical attention. The crisis- or conflict-dominated focus of bioethics supports an understanding of autonomy that does not readily fit the situation of patients with significant functional incapacities whose care needs are often decidedly low-tech and basic. Their situation might seem to fit better under ethical concepts like care or beneficence than autonomy-related concepts like patient rights.[1] Without denying the salience of these concerns, they do not

---

[1] There has been a great deal of recent work on autonomy that criticizes mainstream liberal approaches to the concept for their over-commitment to ideal or abstract understandings or which implicitly embrace questionable theoretical commitments. Recent reformist tendencies cluster around so-called care ethics, feminism, or relationship ethics (see D.E. BUSHNELL (ed.), 'Nagging' Questions: Feminist Ethics in Everyday Life, Lanham, MA, Rowman & Littlefield, 1995; M.A. FINEMAN, The Autonomy Myth: A Theory of Dependency, New York and London, The New Press, 2004; E. FEDER KITTAY & E.K. FEDER, The Subject of Care: Feminist Perspectives on Dependency, Lanham, MA, Rowman & Littlefield, 2002; C. MACKENZIE & N. STOLJAR, Relational Autonomy: Feminist Perspectives on Autonomy, Agency, and the Social Self, New York and Oxford, Oxford University Press, 2000; N. NODDINGS, Caring: A Feminine Approach to Ethics and Moral Education, Berkeley, University of California Press, 2005). These approaches differ from earlier treatments of autonomy by stressing the importance of human development, social interdependence, and affective relationships as central features of ethics and, in some cases, of autonomous agency rather than independence and the capacity for rational decision making. The reassessment of autonomy that I propose incorporates many of these points, but I have eschewed embracing these approaches, because the project of addressing autonomy in long-term care seemed to require not a new ethical theory or set of principles, but a *practical* framework to provide guidance for caregivers and for thinking about how the actual autonomy of an impaired adult in long-term care should be respected. In this contribution, I discuss why such a practical framework for thinking about autonomy is needed and why respecting autonomy requires greater attention to the everyday aspects of what actual autonomy involves in long-term care settings. For a good critical discussion of some of the main criticisms of autonomy by (broadly regarded) feminist thinkers, see J. CHRISTMAN, 'Feminism and Autonomy' in D.E. BUSHNELL (ed.), 'Nagging' Questions: Feminist Ethics in Everyday Life, Lanham, MA, Rowman & Littlefield, 1995, pp. 17-39. Christman argues that one can accept that traditional concepts and theories of autonomy need modification without, however, accepting that autonomy as an ideal or value should be eliminated, even though some feminist critics seem to want to achieve that outcome.

squarely address the most difficult ethical problems involved in long-term care, namely, the pervasive erosion of autonomy.[2] Therefore, rather than substitute an ethics of care for an ethics of autonomy, a re-examination of the meaning of autonomy in long-term care is needed.[3] I will return to this point later.

Thus, my target is the myriad day-to-day situations in which dependent adults receive care, as well as the structure of the institutions within which they live. Individuals needing long-term care, especially nursing home care, usually face problems that most adults seldom worry about, such as, control over what and when to eat, sleep or awake, get out of or return to bed, bathe, dress, use a telephone, take a walk, or see friends or family. Most adults seldom worry about these matters, because control over these daily affairs is normally taken-for-granted. For individuals requiring long-term care, however, these and many other types of routine actions are always in question, because their accomplishment needs the cooperation and assistance of others. Other individuals in long-term care suffer from confusion, memory loss, and cognitive or perceptual impairments that can too-easily result in a dismissal of their sense of self and personal sense of agency.[4] The challenging question is how can considerations of autonomy apply in these situations and, of equal importance, what practical guidance can the appeal to autonomy provide for these elusive situations.

II.

Autonomy is a problem in long-term care in ways that extend beyond the classic autonomy-defined issues like informed consent, decision-making capacity, or surrogate decision-making. Focusing

---

[2] C. Lidz et al., *The Erosion of Autonomy in Long-Term Care*, New York, Oxford University Press, 1992.

[3] G. Agich, 'Reassessing Autonomy in Long-Term Care' in *Hastings Center Report* 20(1990)6, pp. 12-17. See also G. Agich, *Autonomy and Long-Term Care*, New York and Oxford, Oxford University Press, 1993; G. Agich, 'Chronic Illness and Freedom' in S.K. Toombs, D. Barnard & R.A. Carson (eds.), *Chronic Illness: From Experience to Policy*, Bloomington, Indiana University Press, 1995, pp. 129-153; G. Agich, *Dependence and Autonomy in Old Age: An Ethical Framework for Long-Term Care*, Cambridge and New York, Cambridge University Press, 2003.

[4] For a dramatic first-person account of this loss of personal autonomy and sense of self, see C. Laird, *Limbo: A Memoir of Life in a Nursing Home by a Survivor*, Novato, CA, Chandler and Sharp, 1979.

primarily on issues surrounding decision-making about medical interventions, the standard approaches do not provide a sufficiently nuanced basis for addressing the challenges that arise in respecting the actual autonomy of adults who need long-term care. To be sure, such individuals have a wide range of medical or health needs that raise the classic bioethical questions of consent and treatment rights. However, beyond these episodic concerns, individuals needing long-term care importantly also require help with basic activities of daily living (ADLs) like bathing, dressing, transferring from bed or chair, walking, eating, toilet use, and grooming[5] and so-called instrumental ADLs like use of the telephone, traveling via car or public transportation, food or clothes shopping, meal preparation, housework, medication use, and management of money[6], functions that most adults routinely take-for-granted. Addressing the ethical aspects associated with meeting these everyday functions is the essential feature of an ethics that is attuned to long-term care, but one that has been most of peripheral interest in bioethics.[7] Illuminating the ethical underpinnings of these interactions constitutes the formidable challenge that any account of autonomy in long-term care must meet if it is to provide practical guidance.

I have argued that a sufficiently nuanced phenomenological clarification of the structures through which autonomy is actually manifested in the everyday world of social life is needed to provide an autonomy-defined framework of sufficient complexity and can have practical implications for reframing the ethics of long-term care.[8] Such an account develops the concept of *actual autonomy* that Onora O'Neill has introduced into bioethics.[9] Unlike standard treatments of autonomy that typically abstract from the complex details of everyday action and focus primarily on the ethics of decision-making

[5] GILL *et al.*, 'Assessing Risk for the Onset of Functional Dependence among Older Adults: The Role of Physical Performance' in *Journal of the American Geriatrics Society* 43(1995), pp. 603-609.

[6] M. P. LAWTON & E.M. BRODY, 'Assessment of Older People: Self-Maintaining and Instrumental Activities of Daily Living' in *Gerontologist* 9(1969), pp. 179-186.

[7] R.A. KANE & A.L. CAPLAN (eds.), *Everyday Ethics: Resolving Dilemmas in Nursing Home Life*, New York, Springer, 1990.

[8] G. AGICH, 'Reassessing Autonomy in Long-Term Care'; G. AGICH, *Autonomy and Long-Term Care*; G. AGICH, *Dependence and Autonomy in Old Age*.

[9] O. O'NEILL, 'Paternalism and Partial Autonomy' in *Journal of Medical Ethics* 10(1984), pp. 173-179.

conflicts or the nature of autonomy, the concept of *actual autonomy* points in a different direction toward the concrete conditions under which agents act and interact in the everyday world.[10] To understand actual autonomy, then, one must focus on the particularities of the agent, the agent's concrete condition, and the circumstances of their everyday engagements with the world and other persons. The development of this account is motivated by the practical need to center attention on the ethics of day-to-day caring for adults whose functional capacities are compromised or effaced. Although I cannot review this analysis here, I will make a few points about the importance of these structures for understanding actual autonomy in order to show their practical relevance for clinical ethics.

Actual Autonomy

One difficulty with focusing on actual autonomy is the rather messy incompleteness and uncertainty that this phenomenon presents when compared with ideal autonomy. We are forced to say something definite about specific expressions of autonomy in actual cases. We cannot simply rely on hypothetical examples. The problem is that actual autonomy is developmentally and socially conditioned, so that determinate expressions of autonomy will be unique and contextually situated, thus making generalizations unreliable.

"Autonomy," as everyone knows, literally means "self-rule", that is, behavior that is spontaneous and self-initiated. Such behavior is regarded as action in that sense that it manifests intentionality. Action, in turn, can be regarded as free if the individual agent can identify with the elements from which it flows; an action (or choice) is not free or coerced if the agent cannot identify with or dissociates herself from the elements which generate or prompt it.[11] This means that the ability to identify with the constituents of an action is prior to freedom and that autonomy is best understood on the basis of the possession of an identity or of a self having a determinate nature and character. Saying this, of course, does not mean that the self is immutable, but

---

[10] G. AGICH, *Dependence and Autonomy in Old Age*, pp. 83-124.

[11] F. BERGMANN, *On Being Free*, Notre Dame, IN, University of Notre Dame Press, 1977.

that identifications necessarily underlie the true expressions of autonomy.[12] Expressions of autonomy are thus the playing out of who the
individual is as well as who the individual is becoming. The field or
stage for such "playing out" or enactment is the social world of everyday life.

Because autonomous individuals are situated in concrete social
contexts, choice is always contextual and there are always costs associated with any choice. The making of explicit choices or decisions,
however, is not the central feature of our lives; most of our lives are
spent acting in ways that are not experienced as the result of explicit
decision making. Such actions might be taken to be not free on the
traditional view of autonomy, but they are truly autonomous to the
extent that they are consistent with one's identity. In point of fact,
however, in daily life we seem to proceed oblivious to our own spontaneity and freedom. This relative absence of explicit reflective
awareness does not imply that people ordinarily lack autonomy, but
that theoretical accounts of autonomy abstract rather far from its concrete circumstances. The apparent rarity of fully rational and reflective deliberation regarding courses of action and outcomes should
rather remind us of the idealized status of this model of human
autonomy.

The identifications that underlie actual autonomy are not bedrock
stable. Actual autonomy is more like an island in the process of being
formed by submerged volcanic action. Identifications and the autonomy they support are in development as individuals interact with
the world and other persons in the very course of their living, with
some features solidly established above the surface. Paradoxically,
the bulk of a person's everyday autonomy is submerged like an ice-
berg. These hidden aspects of autonomy are most in need of attention
in long-term care, because they are often at issue as the burdens of
care place the integrity of the person at risk. These submerged
aspects of actual autonomy coalesce around four central structures of
the social world of everyday life namely affectivity, communication,
spatiality, and temporality. I have discussed these structures in other
work[13] and need not repeat this detailed analysis here, except to say

---

[12] D. SHOEMAKER, 'Caring, Identification and Agency' in *Ethics* 114(2003), pp. 88-
118.

[13] G. AGICH, *Autonomy and Long-Term Care*; G. AGICH, *Dependence and Autonomy in
Old Age*.

why these structures constitute a practical framework for thinking about what is involved in respecting the actual autonomy of adults who need chronic care.

Thus, to speak of individuals as autonomous requires that we pay attention to the kinds of things with which individuals identify in their lives. Saying this is to expand on the slogan *respect for persons* in a way that reflects the specificity and incorporates the dynamic features of individual life. To respect persons properly requires that we attend to their concrete individuality, to their affective and personal experiences. We need to learn how to acknowledge their habits and identifications if we are to respect their actual autonomy.[14]

Respect for autonomy therefore arguably requires a serious consideration of who the person actually is. That cannot be accomplished from on high, but only in the social world where the accuracy or success of one's interpretation and communication are never fully assured.

World of Everyday Life

Persons live their lives in the shared world of everyday life and their personal autonomy emerges and has its terminus therein. To say that sociality is an essential feature of being a person is to make a descriptive claim about human existence. As such it does not establish an ethic, but it does provide a reference point for articulating what must

---

[14] This is hardly a new point. Mill, too, insisted that individuals require different conditions for their development: "If a person possesses any tolerable amount of common sense and experience, his own mode of existence is the best, not because it is the best in itself, but because it is his own mode. Human beings are not like sheep; and even sheep are not undistinguishably alike. A man cannot get a coat or a pair of boots to fit him unless they are either made to his measure or he has a whole warehouseful to choose from; and is it easier to fit him with a life than with a coat, or are human beings more like one another in their whole physical and spiritual conformation than in the shape of their feet? If it were only that people have diversities of taste, that is reason enough for not attempting to shape them all after one model. But different persons also require different conditions for their spiritual development; and can no more exist healthfully in the same moral than all the varieties of plants can in the same physical atmosphere and climate" (in J.S. MILL, *On Liberty*, Indianapolis, IN, Hackett Publishing Co., 1972, pp. 64-65). For a recent treatment of the constitutive function that identifications play in autonomy, see D. SHOEMAKER, 'Caring, Identification, and Agency' in *Ethics* 114(2003), pp. 88-118.

be considered in respecting autonomy in everyday situations and, by extension, a framework for thinking about autonomy in long-term care.[15] Sociality and the structures of the world of everyday life define the background for agency and the scaffolding for actual manifestations of autonomy. The everyday world is an important context within which to locate actual autonomy, because the everyday world is itself a practical world of doing. It forms what Alfred Schutz has termed the *paramount reality* within which our lives are lived and which provides content that all practical reflection seeks to clarify.[16] The social world of everyday life provides not only the context for the question of how the autonomy of a dependent adult is to be respected, but structural features that define what autonomy *actually* means, because as Egon Bittner has pointed out, "It is impossible to overestimate the *centrality of the subject* for the phenomenal constitution of this world of everyday life".[17]

As subjects in the everyday world, we function on the basis of abilities, habits, and skills acquired historically. Although each person

[15] In many treatments of autonomy, sociality is either left in the background or does not receive explicit attention. It has, however, been given normative prominence in communitarian thought. Communitarianism views sociality as a guide to a distinctive ethic, an ethic that stresses human relationships, commitment, and tradition as central values and as the source for normative ideals. Communitarianism thus elevates the community over the individual. Autonomy as an ideal of the isolated, abstract decision-maker obviously has no place in such a scheme, but the individual as a source of value is also marginalized, if not denied. As a general theory of human nature that denies the importance of shared commitments, the liberal view of autonomy is surely suspect, but views that stress the collective or community over the individual are also suspect. Community and tradition provide no unassailable source for value. Of course, the critics of liberalism are correct in pointing out its deficiencies as an ethical theory. These deficiencies, however, do not invalidate the importance of autonomy within the compass not only of politics and public life, but ethics as well. Thus, distinguishing the liberal view of autonomy as a theory of human nature and a theory of politics is crucial. One can preserve the distinctive contribution of liberal thought to modern culture and society, namely, its protection of individuals from the intrusive power of the state and other individuals as well as its enhancement of the status of persons, while at the same time acknowledging that this view presents at best a truncated understanding of the nature of persons, moral obligation, and ethics without succumbing to the totalizing tendency of communitarian thought that tends to marginalize the importance of individual autonomy.

[16] A. SCHUTZ, *Collected Papers, II: Studies in Social Theory*, ed. A. BRODERSEN, The Hague, Martinus Nijhoff, 1971, pp. 226-229; 341-344.

[17] E. BITTNER, 'Objectivity and Realism in Sociology' in G. PSATHAS (ed.), *Phenomenological Sociology*, New York, Wiley, pp. 119-120.

experiences the world from the perspective of a unique develop-
mental history, the social world of everyday life is shared with and
shaped by others. The underlying view of the person as an agent in
the everyday world thus involves the recognition that the world is
shared and that action and experience are essentially embodied and
subject to the conditions of an embodied existence.[18] This means that
actual autonomy must be understood not only in terms of the mental processes of deliberation and choice, but also in terms of its
embodiment in the shared and historical world of everyday life.

Everyday experience strongly suggests that when there are no obstacles, failures, problems, or difficulties, people are simply busy and
unreflectively bound up with their habitual actions or usual involvement with the world and things. In these circumstances, autonomy is
submerged as effort is suspended.[19] Typically, it is only when routines
break down, when normal expectations are frustrated, or when relationships come undone that reflection and explicit choice really enter.
At those times, we try to deal with new circumstances and in trying
we fall back on the core feature of autonomy. In trying, effort and suffering are involved. These features are recognizable by others and are
a sure sign that the agent in question is minimally autonomous.[20]

III.

A common approach to this question, of course, is that autonomy
ideally restrains the paternalistic motivations that are, or might be,
endemic in meeting the demands of care, but, at most, that tells us
what not to do. If respect for autonomy is to provide practical guidance, it should serve as a positive or directional signpost for guiding
interactions with patients and not just detour us around well-known

---

[18] M. JOHNSON, *The Body in the Mind and the Bodily Basis of Meaning, Imagination,
and Reason*, Chicago, University of Chicago Press, 1987; M. MERLEAU-PONTY, *The
Phenomenology of Perception*, trans. C. SMITH, London, Routledge & Kegan Paul, 1962;
M. MERLEAU-PONTY, *The Structure of Behavior*, trans. A.L. FISHER, Boston, MA, Beacon
Press, 1967.

[19] F. BERGMANN, *On Being Free*, pp. 41-53.

[20] L. HAWORTH, *Autonomy: An Essay in Philosophical Psychology and Ethics*, New
Haven, CT, Yale University Press, 1986; R.M. ZANER, *The Context of Self: A Phenomenological Inquiry Using Medicine as a Clue*, Athens, OH, Ohio University Press, 1981.

problems. A caregiver should be told not just to care for a dependent adult in the abstract, but helped to know how to identify and respect the individuality of the individual receiving the care. Thus, a recitation of the individual's rights will not provide sufficient guidance in answering the caregiver's concern about how to interact with the dependent person so as to respect the person's concrete autonomy. That is, the concept of autonomy has to do more than provide a justification for action; it has to outline the form and quality of actions that comprise respect for autonomy. The practical requirement in clinical ethics is that the appeal to respect autonomy must inform the care giving actions themselves.

Although dependent on others, individuals requiring long-term care are typically active centers of experience and not passive recipients of care. In point of fact, there is considerable give and take in the provision of care. Cooperation is an essential element in effective care giving that involves complex interactions and communication, which already point to a core feature of actual autonomy mentioned above, namely, the effort and suffering of the individual needing care. Ethnographic studies of long-term care have shown that despite their functional incapacities, many patients can importantly help to define the care received.[21] The tendency to marginalize attention to the residual capacities of the recipient of care is unfortunately quite common not only in practice, but in philosophical reflection on care giving as well.

Diemut Grace Bubeck, for example, defines 'caring for' as

> the meeting of the needs of one person by another person where face-to-face interaction between the one who provides care and one who receives care is a crucial element of the overall activity and where the need is of such a nature that it cannot possibly be met by the person in need herself.[22]

---

[21] See, for example, T. DIAMOND, 'Social Policy and Everyday Life in Nursing Homes: A Critical Ethnography' in *Social Science and Medicine* 23(1986), pp. 1287-95; J.F. GUBRIUM, *Living and Dying at Murray Manor*, New York, St. Martin Press, 1975; LIDZ *et al.*, *The Erosion of Autonomy*; J.S. SAVISHINSKY, *The Ends of Time: Life and Work in a Nursing Home*, New York, Bergin & Garvey, 1991; R.R. SHIELD, *Uneasy Endings: Daily Life in an American Nursing Home*, Ithaca and London, Cornell University Press, 1988.

[22] D.G. BUBECK, 'Justice and the Labor of Care' in E. FEDER KITTAY & E.K. FEDER (eds.), *The Subject of Care: Feminist Perspectives on Dependency*, Lanham, MA, Rowman & Littlefield, 2002, p. 163.

This definition importantly recognises the interpersonal and communicative character of caring for, but the primary direction of her analysis is to explore misunderstandings and injustices associated with the role of caregiver rather than to reflect on the nature of mutuality that is implicit in her notion of caring for. Hence, her definition is underdetermined, because how the goal of caring for is defined is not addressed. One cannot say that the goal of care is the caring or the care that is delivered since that would be circular. Saying that the care is given in a face-to-face situation is on the right track, but since even face-to-face care can be delivered in ways that take no regard of the vital needs or identifications of the individual who receives the services that make up the caring, the actual autonomy of the receiver of care might easily be overlooked. Consideration of actual autonomy requires that care giving be defined in such a way that it belongs to the individual receiving it and incorporates that individual's own identifications, if not the individual's own self-determination. Saying the care is delivered face-to-face leaves the most important part implicit.

Characterizing the process of respecting actual autonomy has proven difficult. There is a strong tendency to appeal to a single model or paradigm and to rest the case on that basis. One paradigm that is frequently invoked is the mother-child relationship. It is misleading in a way that illustrates the complexity of the question. Nell Noddings has written that:

> When my infant riddles with delight as I bathe or feed him, I am aware of no burden but only a special delight of my own... Many of the "demands" of caring are not felt as demands. They are, rather, the occasions that offer most of what makes life worth living.[23]

That is undoubtedly true. In a similar vein, Timothy Diamond, an ethnographer who studied nursing homes, reported that one nursing assistant, whom he interviewed, said in all seriousness that "Some shit don't stink" in discussing how she can overcome the difficulties associated with the very hard work of a nursing assistant in meeting the daily needs of dependent adults. When asked to explain what she meant, she replied:

---

[23] N. NODDINGS, *Caring*, p. 52.

It depends on if you like 'em and they like you, and if you know 'em pretty well; it's hard to clean somebody new, or somebody you don't like. If you like 'em, it's like your baby.[24]

We can accept the report of her feeling as accurate without accepting the explanation or model that it implies. While appeal to the mother-child paradigm and the positive affectivity involved in care giving seems so natural, it is dangerous to over-generalize either the mother-child relationship or the affective component as providing a normative guide for long-term care.

Adults are unlike very young children in that their identity and sense of self is far more developed than an infant or young child. Hence, the mutuality of the care giving relationship with dependent adults occurs at more complex levels of communication that are not analogous to the paradigmatic mother-infant relationship and not reducible to affective states akin to maternal affection. This is not to deny that the demands of care may be easier to meet if there is an affective bond, but respecting the actual autonomy of a person cannot rest on such an insecure foundation, because one might feel positively toward the adult receiving care without taking notice of the person's identifications. Failing to do so is apparently quite common in long-term care if the complaints about the perfunctory or depersonalized nature of services provided are true.

Saying this is not to deny the importance of emotional attachment in long-term care. The affective relationship between caregiver and dependent adult is undoubtedly crucial to good care. Without affective engagement, it would be difficult to hold an adult as she gasps for air struggling to breathe and fearing that it might be the end, clean someone as you witness her own shame, or laugh with a demented or confused old person to help her maintain some modicum of social contact. Even routine activities, such as feeding or brushing teeth involve affective connections between caregiver and the person being cared for that can easily be overlooked and undervalued as the stress on technical service and tasks impersonalizes care to the point where bureaucratic efficiency replaces any vestige of personal significance for these basic acts of care. Nonetheless, while the affective component is structurally important in delivering care for a dependent adult, it cannot provide the ground for respecting the person who receives the care.

---

[24] T. DIAMOND, *Social Policy in Everyday Life*, p. 1292.

Unlike an infant, the dependent adult, even if significantly compromised, is usually fully the *subject* of care with an intact identity
and still capable of expressing that identity. It is a subjectivity not
being called forth as in the infant-mother relationship[25], but a subjectivity — perhaps with deficiencies that the caregiver must deal
with, to be sure — that asks to be respected. The concept of actual
autonomy helps here precisely because it directs attention to the
identity and individuality of the person receiving the care as well as
to the interpersonal context within which the care occurs.

Affectivity and communication in the caregiving relationship
remain important as structural elements, but do not define the goal
or meaning of care. Rather they point to the conditions in and
through which the subjectivity of the person is to be identified
through an attunement with the other.[26] In this shared experience, the
actual autonomy of the dependent adult is sounded through a
process of communication that is like the mother-child relationship in
that the care is directed toward the dependent adult, but unlike it in
that the dependent adult determines the meaningfulness of the care
received.

Actual Autonomy in Long-Term Care

The practical implications of a turn to actual autonomy for long-term
care are important. Respect for autonomy cannot mean that caregivers are primarily and absolutely precluded from influencing the
decisions of dependent adults. To be exposed to influence, especially
influence that aims at the individual's own sense of well-being, does
not violate autonomy. The interpersonal relationship between the
receiver of care and caregiver is far more complicated, especially in
long-term care, than the worrisome model of medical paternalism

---

[25] J. BOWLBY, *Attachment and Loss: Volume I, Attachment*, New York, Basic Books,
1969; R. SPITZ, *The First Year of Life*, New York, International University Press, 1965.

[26] Alfred Schutz has characterized the phenomenon in a paper entitled, "Making
Music Together" (A. SCHUTZ, *Collected Papers*, pp. 159-78) as a "mutual tuning-in" during which each individual contributes to the definition of the shared experience. *Making music together* involves the sharing of one's inner or subjective time, because when
people make music together they come to inhabit the same stream of time, and so the
mutual tuning-in relationship is really a constituting of intersubjectivity, a concept
that Schutz popularized as a middle way between objectivity and subjectivity.

that dominates bioethical thinking. In long-term care, especially where care is provided by family or by paid caregivers in the patient's home, the dependent adult can retain significant power and independence, especially in regards to the caregiver. This is not to deny that the autonomy of frail old people can readily succumb to over zealous ministrations, but this is where the attention to actual autonomy gains its practical edge. By making actual autonomy the focus of respect, the attention is shifted to the concrete individual and away from abstractions that prevent the caregiver from establishing a truly interpersonal connection.

The interpersonal relationships that develop between dependent adults and caregivers are far more relevant for ethical analysis than the professional power or authority that the critique of medical paternalism seeks to curb. Focusing on actual autonomy highlights a range of difficult practical concerns about long-term care arrangements that would otherwise be overlooked. For example, respecting autonomy by expanding choices can be undertaken without attention to whether the choices actually afforded are meaningful or worth making for the individuals themselves.[27] Even when individuals are afforded an array of choices, autonomy may not be meaningfully enhanced if the choices are not meaningful for them. Enlarging the range of meal choices for an individual who observes ethically or religiously based dietary restrictions, for example, does not necessarily augment autonomy in a meaningful way. Unless the options are consistent with the particular dietary preferences that are meaningful in the person's way of life, they simply increase the burden of choice.

Consider the typical kinds of choices that are afforded individuals in nursing homes — choices regarding limited outings, the use of special services like hair dressing, participation in structured social and recreational activities like bingo, or choosing when and what to eat, with whom to associate, or "permission" to ask or not ask staff for help. No matter how extensive this list is, it is seldom considered whether the choices are meaningful for the individuals themselves. However, if the alternatives available do not preserve or enhance the

---

[27] As Gerald Dworkin put it: "What does have intrinsic value is not having choices but being recognized as a kind of creature who is capable of making choices." G. DWORKIN, *The Theory and Practice of Autonomy*, Cambridge, Cambridge University Press, 1988, p. 80.

unique individuality and identity of the persons being cared for, then the choices are not consistent with actual autonomy and might actually impede its expression.

Consider the seventy-five year old woman whose own health is deteriorating. She must make difficult decisions regarding the care of her seventy-eight year old husband, who has suffered a stroke and is now bedridden. Similarly, the husband must accept institutionalization or watch as his own care literally consumes his wife. The family of such a couple, too, must struggle with choices that are equally difficult. Do they take the couple into their households for care? Do they separate the couple and arrange for different types or locations of care for each of their parents? Sometimes, the cost to self for a parent to live with his or her children is too great not because the parent fears a loss of independence, but because the parent cannot identify with the burden placed on the children or the loss of friends and familiar surroundings. The psychological consequence of this point is evident everywhere in long-term care. Non-identification characteristically carries with it a sense of passivity that is evident in withdrawal and generalized depression that is often seen in institutionalized old people.[28]

---

[28] This is most forcefully seen in old people whose incapacities involve or require extended bed rest.

"After several days, the bed begins to smell. The odors of cloth, bed sheets, covers, pillows, and pajamas become an intimate and prominent part of the limited world of the sick person. The existence of the individual becomes vapid and stale as the patient slips into passivity and dependence. Since others must do things, the individual loses physical contact not only with the surroundings, but also with one's own body. Daily hygiene and other activities of daily living are taken over by others; one's usual privacy is lost. As a result, it seems that nothing is left to the person. It is as if one has abdicated whole portions of the self. The experience of enforced inactivity manifests itself in a psychological distancing from the external world and one's own body." (J. BERGSMA & D. THOMASMA, *Health Care: Its Psychosocial Dimensions*, Pittsburgh, PA, Duquesne University Press, 1982, p. 131)

The idea of movement itself implies a functional relationship between vital interests and values, between behavior and circumstances, between position and a sense of place, between action and things in the world (J. BERGSMA & D. THOMASMA, *Health Care*, p. 131). Hence, the sick or impaired individual experiences normal realities differently. The entire world takes on a sense of being cramped and remote or simply alien. The disabled adult, especially one without significant or meaningful social contacts and interactions, therefore naturally focuses on his own bodily processes creating a very narrow and restricted horizon for experience. The attention to "bed and body work" by caregivers further insinuates a sense of isolation and reinforces and confirms the individual's sense of being lost or confused.

Consider a wheel-chair bound individual being assisted by others in various activities of daily living. This person is devoted to the cause of Food for Peace (FFP). What this person can do for this cause is limited, yet she identifies strongly with it. She stuffs envelops twice a week for the local FFP chapter and rejoices when she sees a television feature on FFP's projects. She has visitors from the FFP organization. Her most meaningful activities are those that relate to FFP. She may not care whether she has her bath at 6:00 a.m. on Thursday or at 2:00 p.m. on Friday. Not all choices matter to her, just those that are meaningful in terms of her participatory identification in a larger project. A similar and more familiar case would be the intense involvement of an elder in her grandchildren or hobby or commitment to a favorite sports team. The inability to shop or leave the home or institution may be far less significant for such an individual than the ability to entertain her family, pursue her hobby, or watch the team compete on television. The central point is that such matters cannot be determined in general, but only specifically in an individual case. At the same time, others needing long-term care focus on their immediate circumstances. For them, the timing of meals, bathing, or bed or freedom of movement within and outside their living space might matter significantly.

Because the spatial environment is such an important facet of actual autonomy, its use to either control elders or enhance their range of experience is an important aspect in respecting the actual autonomy of individuals in long-term care. Electing protection or safety without considering the costs to the quality of experience of the cognitively impaired elder is likely to thwart rather than respect that person's autonomy.[29] Coons[30] suggested that rigid schedules and hospital-like design elements are not suitable for long-term care, particularly for residents who are cognitively impaired, because they need an environment that affords opportunities to express their developed tendencies and habits by affording them a variety of spaces in which to experience the world. Such experiential choices facilitate the

---

[29] B. COLLOPY, 'Safety and Independence: Rethinking Some Basic Concepts in Long-Term Care' in L.D. McCULLOUGH & N.L. WILSON (eds.), *Long-Term Care Decisions: Ethical and Conceptual Dimensions*, Baltimore and London, Johns Hopkins University Press, 1995, pp. 137-152.

[30] D. COONS, *Designing a Residential Care Unit for Persons with Dementia*, Washington, DC, Office of Technology Assessment, 1987.

person's control of her situation. The operative sense of identification understood as the rudiment of autonomous expression thus provides a positive and practical guide for enhancing a range of choices that are meaningful for the confused and cognitively impaired elder. As Cohen and Weisman put it:

> To the extent that individuals have the opportunity to make meaningful decisions about their environments, they can maintain ties to their past lives... For people with dementia, familiar artifacts, activities, and spaces can provide valuable personal associations and can stimulate opportunities for social interaction and meaningful activity.[31]

Thus, attending to actual autonomy can help caregivers to interact with dependent adults in such a way that the adult's identifications are respected as their care needs are met. Robert Kastenbaum has observed that unfortunately in institutional long-term care

> We often see the clinical ambiance minus the clinical benefits. The person who is a patient only temporarily can adjust to the unfamiliar and unlovely hospital routines knowing that this is only an interlude. Some comfort and individuality is sacrificed; however, in fair return the person receives state-of-the-art medical and nursing care. By contrast, the geriatric milieu is a long-term or permanent arrangement for many people, and the clinical ambiance is not counterbalanced by superb care. Perhaps the most infuriating note from the standpoint of the patient is the attitude that "this is all for your own good." It is not—and everybody knows it.[32]

Kastenbaum argues that the necessary goal for a clinical milieu is to make the world right again. Frail and impaired older persons experience many sorrows, losses, fears, and frustrations in addition to the physical ailments and disabilities. Certainly, a therapeutic environment must provide treatments to allay discomfort and help individuals maintain a level of integrated functioning. But there must be a broader environment that is conducive to the well-being of people who need long-term services besides the episodic medical

---

[31] U. COHEN & G.D. WEISMAN, 'Environmental Design to Maximize Autonomy for Older Adults with Cognitive Impairments' in *Generations* 14(1990), p. 76.

[32] R. KASTENBAUM, 'Can the Clinical Milieu Be Therapeutic?' in G.D. ROWLES & R.J. OHTA (eds.), *Aging and Milieu: Environmental Perspectives on Growing Old*, New York, Academic Press, 1983, p. 11.

treatments that are now the focus of care. In effect, geriatric practice must attend to what Hans Selye has classically termed "the syndrome of just being sick", that is to say the pervasive sense that things are just not right.[33] Besides specific disabilities and pains, there is a sense of the world gone awry, a pervasive sense of loss or what might be simply termed *existential despair*. Kastenbaum argues that the just being sick syndrome can be countered effectively by a milieu that develops a systematic and encompassing framework of positive expectations on the part of everyone involved. Clarifying the components of such a milieu would be one way to make the respect for autonomy practical in long-term care. To do that, however, requires that the concept of autonomy be re-conceptualized along the lines suggested above.

Conclusion

The turn to actual, as opposed to ideal, autonomy is needed in long-term care, because the conditions of dependence that necessitate chronic care and the mundane interactions that make up chronic care otherwise fall outside standard applications of autonomy. Because actual autonomy views the person as a developed individual in concrete relationships with others and within the everyday world of social action, it provides a framework for re-thinking the practices and the social and institutional arrangements associated with long-term care. In doing so, autonomy in long-term care illustrates the salience of autonomy for clinical ethics across a range of concerns.

References

AGICH, G.J., 'Reassessing Autonomy in Long-Term Care' in *Hastings Center Report* 20(1990)6, pp. 12-17.

AGICH, G.J., *Autonomy and Long-Term Care*, New York and Oxford, Oxford University Press, 1993.

AGICH, G.J., 'Chronic Illness and Freedom' in S.K. TOOMBS, D. BARNARD & R.A. CARSON (eds.), *Chronic Illness: From Experience to Policy*, Bloomington, Indiana University Press, 1995, pp. 129-153.

---

[33] H. SELYE, *The Stress of Life*, New York, McGraw-Hill, 1956.

AGICH, G.J., *Dependence and Autonomy in Old Age: An Ethical Framework for Long-Term Care*, Cambridge and New York, Cambridge University Press, 2003.

BERGMANN, F., *On Being Free*, Notre Dame, IN, University of Notre Dame Press, 1977.

BERGSMA, J. & D. THOMASMA, *Health Care: Its Psychosocial Dimensions*, Pittsburgh, PA, Duquesne University Press, 1982.

BITTNER, E., 'Objectivity and Realism in Sociology' in G. PSATHAS (ed.), *Phenomenological Sociology*, New York, Wiley, 1973, pp. 109-25.

BOWLBY, J., *Attachment and Loss: Volume I, Attachment*, New York, Basic Books, 1969.

BUBECK, D.G., 'Justice and the Labor of Care' in E. FEDER KITTAY & E.K. FEDER (eds.), *The Subject of Care: Feminist Perspectives on Dependency*, Lanham, MA, Rowman and Littlefield, 2002, pp. 160-185.

BUSHNELL, D.E. (ed.), *'Nagging' Questions: Feminist Ethics in Everyday Life*, Lanham, MA, Rowman & Littlefield, 1995.

CHRISTMAN, J., 'Feminism and Autonomy' in D.E. BUSHNELL (ed.), *'Nagging' Questions: Feminist Ethics in Everyday Life*, Lanham, MD, Rowman & Littlefield, 1995, pp. 17-39.

COLLOPY, B., 'Safety and Independence: Rethinking Some Basic Concepts in Long-Term Care' in L.D. MCCULLOUGH & N.L. WILSON (eds.), *Long-Term Care Decisions: Ethical and Conceptual Dimensions*, Baltimore and London, Johns Hopkins University Press, 1995, pp. 137-52.

COHEN, U. & G.D. WEISMAN, 'Environmental Design to Maximize Autonomy for Older Adults with Cognitive Impairments' in *Generations* 14(1990), pp. 75-78.

COONS, D., *Designing a Residential Care Unit for Persons with Dementia*, Washington, DC, Office of Technology Assessment, 1987.

DIAMOND, T., 'Social Policy and Everyday Life in Nursing Homes: A Critical Ethnography' in *Social Science and Medicine* 23(1986), pp. 1287-95.

DWORKIN, G., *The Theory and Practice of Autonomy*, Cambridge, Cambridge University Press, 1988.

FINEMAN, M.A., *The Autonomy Myth: A Theory of Dependency*, New York and London: The New Press, 2004.

GILL, T.M., C.S. WILLIAMS & M.E. TINETTI, 'Assessing Risk for the Onset of Functional Dependence among Older Adults: The Role of Physical Performance' in *Journal of the American Geriatrics Society* 43(1995), pp. 603-609.

GUBRIUM, J.F., *Living and Dying at Murray Manor*, New York, St. Martin's Press, 1975.

HAWORTH, L., *Autonomy: An Essay in Philosophical Psychology and Ethics*, New Haven, CT, Yale University Press, 1986.

JOHNSON, M., *The Body in the Mind and the Bodily Basis of Meaning, Imagination, and Reason*, Chicago, University of Chicago Press, 1987.

Kane, R.A. & A.L. Caplan (eds.), *Everyday Ethics: Resolving Dilemmas in Nursing Home Life*, New York, Springer, 1990.

Kastenbaum, R., 'Can the Clinical Milieu Be Therapeutic?' in G.D. Rowles & R.J. Ohta (eds.), *Aging and Milieu: Environmental Perspectives on Growing Old*, New York, Academic Press, 1983, pp. 3-15.

Kittay, E.F & E.K. Feder, *The Subject of Care: Feminist Perspectives on Dependency*, Lanham, MA, Rowman and Littlefield, 2002.

Laird, C., *Limbo: A Memoir of Life in a Nursing Home by a Survivor*, Novato, CA, Chandler and Sharp, 1979.

Lawton, M.P. & E.M. Brody, 'Assessment of Older People: Self-Maintaining and Instrumental Activities of Daily Living' in *Gerontologist* 9(1969), pp. 179-186.

Lidz, C.W., L. Fischer & R.M. Arnold, *The Erosion of Autonomy in Long-Term Care*, New York, Oxford University Press, 1992.

Mackenzie, C. & N. Stoljar, *Relational Autonomy: Feminist Perspectives on Autonomy, Agency, and the Social Self*, New York and Oxford, Oxford University Press, 2000.

Merleau-Ponty, M., *The Phenomenology of Perception*, trans. C. Smith, London, Routledge & Kegan Paul, 1962.

Merleau-Ponty, M., *The Structure of Behavior*, trans. A.L. Fisher, Boston, MA, Beacon Press, 1967.

Mill J.S., *On Liberty*, Indianapolis, IN, Hackett Publishing Co., 1972.

Noddings, N., *Caring: A Feminine Approach to Ethics and Moral Education*, Berkeley, University of California Press, 2005.

O'Neill, O., 'Paternalism and Partial Autonomy' in *Journal of Medical Ethics* 10(1984), pp. 173-178.

Savishinsky, J.S., *The Ends of Time: Life and Work in a Nursing Home*, New York, Bergin & Garvey, 1991.

Schutz, A., *The Phenomenology of the Social World* (transl. G. Walsh & F. Lehnert), Evanston, IL, Northwestern University Press, 1967.

Schutz, A., *Collected Papers, II: Studies in Social Theory*, ed. A. Brodersen, The Hague, Martinus Nijhoff, 1971.

Selye, H., *The Stress of Life*, New York, McGraw-Hill, 1956.

Shield, R.R., *Uneasy Endings: Daily Life in an American Nursing Home*, Ithaca and London, Cornell University Press, 1988.

Shoemaker, D., 'Caring, Identification, and Agency' in *Ethics* 114(2003), pp. 88-118.

Spitz, R., *The First Year of Life*, New York, International University Press, 1965.

Zaner, R.M., *The Context of Self: A Phenomenological Inquiry Using Medicine as a Clue*, Athens, OH, Ohio University Press, 1981.

3. AUTONOMY IN DEPENDENCE
A Defence of Careful Solidarity

Yvonne Denier

Medical intervention and medical care aim to restore a patient's autonomy as well as possible, or in cases where such restoration cannot or can no longer be realised, they aim to take care of the person in distress and ease his pain and suffering in the best possible way.

This seemingly simple starting-point includes three issues that deserve careful consideration. The first and most important issue is the idea that autonomy is generally acknowledged as a fundamental value for determining human well-being and the good life. What does this mean? In the first section of this paper, I will examine the typical connections between the values of autonomy, human well-being and the good life. I will do this against the background of the informed consent doctrine, which is well-known in medical ethics. The main questions that I will try to answer here are: what is implied in the normative value of autonomy? In what respects is it a value that is worthy of pursuit? Which forms of normativity are included in the value of autonomy?

In the second section, I will take a closer look at the relationship between medicine and autonomy. Medical intervention and medical care aim at realising autonomy if it was absent before, or at restoring it if it has been affected by illness or accident. I will try to show that the medical relationship between physician and patient reveals that the normative value of autonomy includes a subjective as well as an objective aspect, and that both of these aspects are important elements of a person's health condition. Subsequently, I will examine the implications of this twofold normativity of autonomy in the light of the viewpoint that understands the physician-patient relationship as a relationship of solidarity, i.e. of an alliance characterised by mutual dignity and respect.

In the third section, I will concentrate on the idea that when restoration or realisation of autonomy is not or no longer possible, we ought to take care of the patient concerned as well as possible in order to ensure that his situation of dependence is the best of a bad situation. In doing this however, we must be cautious because of the ambiguity of care. In this final section, I will show how both the subjective and objective normativity of autonomy illustrate the emancipatory function of care as well as the horror of being stuck in dependence. I will also show that the solidarity model is probably the best answer to this ambiguity.

1. Autonomy, Well-Being and the Good Life.

Let us start with the first research question: the connection between the values of autonomy, human well-being and the good life.

Since modernity, autonomy has been generally acknowledged as an important value. The concept of autonomy derives from the Greek *autos* or "self" and *nomos* or "law". At first, the term referred to the self-governance of the Hellenic city-states. Today however, the concept is mainly used for individuals. It refers to a range of normative or value-laden concepts such as privacy, liberty rights, individual choice, self-determination, personal self-governance, et cetera. For example, the Oxford English Dictionary defines autonomy as (1) the right or condition of self-government, (2) freedom of the will and (3) independence, freedom from external control or influence; personal liberty.

Altogether, this means that the *absence of constraint* in decision-making or self-realisation is a necessary condition for autonomy. As professor Beauchamp stresses in his paper, constraint can have an *external* origin (which is the case in matters of coercion by others), or it can have an *internal* source (which is the case in matters of mental incapacity). Analogously, autonomy can be defined according to its external or its internal structure. Let us have a closer look at both these structures of autonomy.

Let us firstly examine the definition of autonomy according to its external structure. According to John Stuart Mill autonomy is related to free action, based on self-interest. The limit is *external*: my freedom is limited by the freedom of others.[1] In this respect, autonomy is a

---

[1] J.S. MILL, *On Liberty*, s.l., Wordsworth, 1859 (ed. 1996).

typical characteristic of the self-determining and self-ruling subject without any reference to a subject-transcending objectivity. As such, it reflects a subjectivistic preference perspective, or hedonism: the autonomous subject acts freely as far as he acts in the light of his own ideas, wishes and preferences. In doing this, he is only limited by the freedom of others.

Contrary to Mill, Immanuel Kant describes the *internal* structure of autonomy. Autonomy of the will, as a condition for moral action, is the ability to act according to principles that can be willed as a universal law. Autonomy as "Selbstgezetzlichkeit des Willens" means, in a negative sense, independence from external determination of the self, by passions and inclinations, and in a positive sense self-determination as "Selbstgesetzgebung."[2] Kant too understands autonomous action as free action, but this freedom is not the subjectivistic freedom to be able to do as one pleases. According to Kant, authentic freedom is freedom to do one's moral duty. As such, autonomy refers to an order which transcends man's subjective wishes and desires.

Although the concept of autonomy is an idea that is a typical characteristic of the period of Enlightenment, it has become prominent in medical ethics only from the second half of the twentieth century. This happened with the tide of growing criticism on the until then dominant *paternalism* in the relationship between physician and patient.

Taking into account the *external* as well as the *internal* constraint of self-determination and self-governance, Beauchamp and Childress define autonomy in their *Principles of Biomedical Ethics* as "Self-rule that is free from both controlling interference by others and from limitations, such as an inadequate understanding, that prevent meaningful choice."[3]

In medical ethics the concept of autonomy is elaborated predominantly in the domain of decision-making in medical treatment, and more specifically in the theories on free and informed consent. In this framework, two concepts are of central importance, that is, the concepts of well-being and autonomy.[4] On the one hand, we may safely

---

[2] I. KANT, *Kritik der praktischen Vernunft*, Hamburg, Meiner, 1990, §8, p. 39; O. HÖFFE, *Immanuel Kant*, München, Beck, 2000, pp. 173-207.

[3] In: T.L. BEAUCHAMP & J.F. CHILDRESS, *The Principles of Biomedical Ethics*, New York, Oxford University Press, 2001, p. 58.

[4] D. BROCK, 'Quality of Life Measures in Health Care and Medical Ethics' in M.C. NUSSBAUM & A. SEN (eds.), *The Quality of Life*, Oxford, Clarendon Press, 1993, pp. 95-132, p.107.

say that it is the informed consent doctrine's ultimate aim to serve and improve the *well-being* of the patient. For the sake of argument, well-being is understood here in the narrow, *physical* sense of being determined by one's objectively determinable mental state, activities and the ability to function. Though at least equally important, on the other hand, is respect for self-determination or *autonomy* of the patient; whereby autonomy is understood as the person-related importance that people attach to forming, revising and pursuing in their choices and actions their own plan of life, according to their own personal conception of the good. Or put in other words, it includes the importance that persons attach to making meaningful choices, which may have an important influence on their lives, such as decisions concerning medical intervention and care, according to their own values.

There is a historical reason to believe that of the two values of *physical well-being* and *autonomy* as self-determination, the value of *autonomy* can be considered as possessing the greatest moral weight. The history of the informed consent doctrine shows that if a patient decides autonomously in favour of a certain action, which is at odds with his physical well-being (for example, a patient with terminal cancer who decides to refuse further chemotherapy), this decision is to be honoured out of respect for the patient's autonomy in making a free and informed decision. Interference with this decision is hard to justify, even with the best of intentions for the patient's physical well-being. In this line of reasoning, one could argue that this viewpoint fully supports Mill's widely known external definition of autonomy:

> "The sole end for which mankind are warranted, individually or collectively, in interfering with the liberty of action of any of their number, is self-protection. That the only purpose for which power can be rightfully exercised over any member of a civilised community, against his will, is to prevent harm to others. His own good, either physical or moral, is not a sufficient warrant. He cannot rightfully be compelled to do or forbear because it will be better for him to do so, because it will make him happier, because, in the opinions of others, to do so would be wise or even right."[5]

Contrary to this view, I believe that a more plausible explanation of the distinctive moral weight of autonomy takes into account the *external* as well as the *internal* definition of autonomy, and this from

[5] J.S. MILL, *On Liberty*, p. 13.

the perspective of a threefold connection between autonomy, well-being and the good life.

The conventional view in medicine (with which I refer to our general, immediate and spontaneous common-sense beliefs about the relationship between autonomy, well-being, and the good life) roughly equalises the patient's physical well-being with the patient's good, and understands individual autonomy as a value independent from the patient's physical well-being or good (cf. Figure 1). This implies that respect for the patient's autonomy sometimes justifies respecting choices in medical treatment that go against the patient's physical well-being, paternalistically understood as the patient's good.[6] That is why we, at first sight, may find it hard to understand and to accept that a patient decides autonomously in favour of a certain action or intervention, which is at odds with his physical well-being. At first sight, we may be inclined to think "This is not good for you. This cannot be your true choice." Our spontaneous reaction may be "Are you really sure about this?" There appears to be a conflict between various conceptions of what that patient's good is.

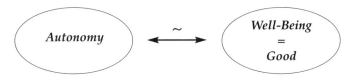

Figure 1: the Conventional View[7]

In contrast however, autonomy is also generally understood as a concept, which reflects the recognition of the individual as a person who is capable of forming his own concept of the good life. The good life is broadly understood then as including one's particular values concerning one's life plans, expectations regarding the good life, happiness, freedom, beauty, identity, quality et cetera. If respect for autonomy is a fundamental value, fundamental in the sense of being included in the idea of respect for the human person, then it is reasonable to interpret the capacity for forming a conception of the good

---

[6] The conventional view can be found in the independent principles of 'beneficence' and 'autonomy' in T.L. BEAUCHAMP & J.F. CHILDRESS, *The Principles of Biomedical Ethics*, 2001.

[7] The ~ refers to a relation of agreement; the ↔ to the possibility of conflict.

life as being *part* of autonomy, rather than considering both autonomy and the good as independent values, potentially in conflict with each other.

The same goes, I believe, for physical well-being. In an important sense, autonomy as self-governance not only includes the idea of *mental capacity* to form one's plan of action free from external constraint, but also the idea of *independent action* understood as the biological or functional capacity to actually physically *carry out* one's plan of action.

As the Spanish film *Mar Adentro* shows, the idea of autonomy as self-rule becomes a meagre concept if it does not take the idea of bodily or functional autonomy into account.[8] The film depicts the real-life story of the Spaniard Ramon Sanpedro who, after a diving accident, spends his life in a paralysed state. He is fully paralysed up to his neck. One aspect of the film, which is particularly interesting, is that Ramon Sanpedro at a certain moment says that being in a state of extreme physical dependence is a true infringement of one's freedom, privacy and autonomy. This is interesting in two ways. On the one hand, because you literally cannot carry out what you wish to do, you constantly need help. This situation is comparable to the liberty of the frustrated slave, which has been analysed in Thomas Nys's contribution: "The frustrated slave who is free to have all the wishes and dreams he can imagine while, at the same time, he sees himself shackled in chains and locks. This is autonomy captured in tears; freedom expressed in the dull sounds of fists banging on prison walls."[9] The point of comparison is that the prison walls can be one's own body, when in a state of full paralysis. On the other hand, because of this situation of extreme dependence in which you constantly need help to carry out your life, you often need to defend yourself against some of the best intentions of the care-givers who think that they know, better than yourself, which plans of action serve your interests best; which plans of action serve your good.

Against this background, and in order to show that there is an important physical aspect of autonomy as well, I have previously defined well-being expressly as *physical* well-being, understood in the narrow, functional sense of being determined by mental state, activities and the ability to function. Along the lines of the following arguments,

---

[8] *Mar Adentro (The Sea Inside)*, directed by Alejandro Amenábar, 2004.
[9] See the contribution of Thomas Nys in this volume.

I will gradually develop a clearer view on the way in which the three values of autonomy, physical well-being and the good are connected.

First of all, it is important to note that the threefold connection that I wish to make between autonomy, physical well-being and the good life introduces a difference between the good life for a person and that person's physical well-being, in the sense that individual self-determination *in the light of* one's particular conception of the good life may come into conflict with one's physical well-being (as I have visualised in Figure 2). Dan Brock correspondingly defines autonomy as a central aspect of the good life:

> "It is in the exercise of self-determination that we maintain some control over, and take responsibility for, our lives and for what we will become. This is not to deny, of course, that there are always substantial limits and constraints within which we must exercise this judgement and choice. But it is to say that showing respect for people through respecting their self-determination acknowledges the fundamental place of self-determination in a good life."[10]

According to this viewpoint, the *external* determination of autonomy takes into account external legitimate and illegitimate limits and restrictions, connected to *physical* well-being. The *internal* structure takes into consideration *self-determination* in connection with the *good life*.

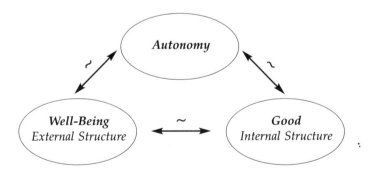

Figure 2: The Threefold Model

Against the background of this threefold connection between autonomy, well-being and the good life, one can understand that within

---

[10] D. BROCK, 'Quality of Life Measures in Health Care and Medical Ethics' 1993, pp. 109-110.

his conception of the good life a person can make a free and deliberate choice to reduce his own physical well-being, for example for the well-being of others. An example of this would be a parent who saves their child's life by choosing to donate a kidney or a piece of their liver for transplantation.

Inversely, but less problematic from the medical point of view, it is possible that a person autonomously takes certain decisions in favour of his physical well-being, which run counter to his conception of the good life. An example of this would be the couple that chooses to abandon its wish for a second child because the health risks for the mother have turned out to be too great. Another example would be the true gourmet who suffers from diabetes and decides to stick to his diet even though this means that he is no longer able to enjoy his most favourite dish.

With the requirement to respect the patient's choice the informed consent doctrine implies that the best life for a person is a life of self-determination and individual choice, even if this leads to a reduction of this person's physical well-being or his experience of the good life.

Additionally, it is important to note that this definition of autonomy does not entail an *ontological* statement, providing a determination of the essence of humanity. Advocates of the ideology of self-sufficiency might perhaps support an ontological characterisation of the autonomy concept, but this soon ends up in absurdity.[11] For it would entail that people who are not or no longer autonomous, like for instance premature babies or patients suffering from Alzheimer's disease, are actually not truly human beings. For Kant however, human dignity resides in the *possibility or capacity* for autonomy.

The threefold model does imply however, that autonomy has an important *normative* value in the light of what it means to be human. Respect for the autonomy of a human being is a moral demand and implies that everyone ought to be able to fully develop his capacity for autonomy. In hedonistic theories and preference theories this normative value of autonomy is implemented in a subjective way. Autonomy is defined then as the possibility to pursue freely and deliberately what one finds enjoyable or what one wishes or prefers.

---

[11] The background of this position is amongst others the discussion Charles Taylor enters into in *Sources of the Self*, with the so-called 'modern naturalist consciousness', which understands the essence of human identity as being independent and 'self-sufficient'. See C. TAYLOR, *Sources of the Self. The Making of the Modern Identity*, Cambridge, Harvard University Press, 1989.

The objective normativity of autonomy is supported by so-called, and I borrow this term from Derek Parfit, 'ideal theories', which equalise the value of autonomy with the personal realisation of objective, normative ideals such as reasonableness and freedom.[12]

As Parfit suggests in appendix I of his *Reasons and Persons*, Philosophical literature and debate exhibit a strong tendency to emphasise one position at the expense of the other. For the hedonistic view and preference theory, a particular object or situation is part of the good life only insofar as it rends pleasure or satisfies preferences. In the position of 'ideal theory' normative ideals are an essential part of the good life. Whether or not the person involved *enjoys* himself more or *prefers* to achieve those ideals is of no importance. Accordingly, ideal theorists consider hedonism and preference theory as loose enjoyment theory, whereas hedonists and supporters of preference theory consider ideal theory to be formal and empty.

In the following two sections, I will try to show that there is no need whatsoever to reduce the subjective and objective normativity of autonomy to either plain enjoyment and preference satisfaction, or to the pursuit of formal and empty normative ideals. As will become clear, the above-defended threefold connection between autonomy, physical well-being and the good life plays an important role in this argument. The way in which these concepts function within the physician-patient relationship and in situations of sheer dependence and need, clarifies that a valuable *combination rather than a mutual execration* of both the objective and subjective normativity of autonomy is necessary to reach a clear understanding of what happens in such situations of sheer dependence and need.

2. Autonomy and Medical Intervention

Let us now take a closer look at the relationship between medicine and autonomy. The definition of autonomy as including objective as well as a subjective normativity can be derived from the function and goal, which is ascribed to medicine and to medical decision-making.

Against the background of a Cartesian dualistic context, some scientists defend a naturalistic and functionalistic conception of medicine. According to this view, the sole end of medicine is the promo-

---

[12] In: D. PARFIT, *Reasons and Persons*, Oxford, Clarendon Press, 1984, pp. 493-502.

tion and protection of health and the healthy person. Happiness, desires or preferences are not included in the mission of medicine. According to the naturalistic view, health is a characteristic of individual biological organisms, the components of which have specific functions that aim at the preservation and functioning of the organic whole. Health is nothing more than proper functioning of the components. As Leon Kass puts it:

> "Health is a natural standard or norm — not a moral norm, not a 'value' as opposed to a 'fact', not an obligation — a state of being that reveals itself in activity as a standard of bodily excellence or fitness."[13]

Put in other words, health and illness are positive and negative biological-functional quantities, and as a scientist the physician is the only proper judge of whether or not someone is healthy and which therapeutic interventions are best called for in the latter case. Following Deleuze and Guattari, the philosopher Nick Fox refers to this view as "the modern discourse of biomedicine" which approaches a person as a "body-with-organs":

> "[Biomedicine describes] the body in terms of function as related to form. When functioning adequately (according to norms set by the discourse), it is in a state of 'health', deviations are defined as 'illness', to be treated and perhaps cured by those expert in the discipline of biomedicine — doctors."[14]

The severely criticised paternalism, in which the doctor as a scientific authority takes medical decisions on the basis of the idea that he alone knows what serves best the patient's interests, without taking into account the patient's personal wishes, conceptions and convic-

---

[13] In: L. KASS, *Towards a More Natural Science*, New York, Free Press, 1985, p. 173. See also: A.L. CAPLAN, (et al.), *Concepts of Health and Disease: Interdisciplinary Perspectives*, Reading, Addison-Wesley, 1981; C. BOORSE, 'On the Distinction between Health and Disease' in *Philosophy and Public Affairs* 5(1975), pp. 49-68; K. DIERICKX, *Genetisch gezond? Ethische en sociale aspecten van genetische tests en screenings* [Genetically Healthy? Ethical and Social Aspects of Genetic Tests and Screenings], Antwerpen, Intersentia, 1999.

[14] In: N. FOX, 'Postmodernism and Health' in A. PETERSEN & C. WADDELL (eds.), *Health Matters: A Sociology of Illness, Prevention and Care*, Buckingham, Open University Press, 1998, pp. 9-22, p. 13. See also: G. DELEUZE & F. GUATTARI, *Anti-Oedipus: Capitalism and Schizophrenia*, London, Athlone, 1984. The naturalistic and functionalistic conception of medicine is severely criticised in Herman De Dijn's *De herontdekking van de ziel. Voor een volwaardige kwaliteitszorg* [The Rediscovery of the Soul. Towards a Full Quality Care.], Nijmegen, Valkhof Pers, 1999.

tions, is founded on a naturalistic view on medicine. Within the naturalistic discourse, paternalism serves the power and expertise of the medical profession. The value of medical action is judged unilaterally on the success of the action, which can be assessed in an objective-biological way. The patient's autonomy plays no part, and neither does his personal conception of the good life. An objective normativity is attributed only to the patient's physical and biological well-being. According to this view, care for the physical well-being of a patient in need is an ethical demand and the sole duty of medicine.

Conversely, it is reasonable to believe that the Cartesian dualism of naturalistic medicine comes to the surface in another shape, that is, when the principle of autonomy is translated in the radical right to self-determination of the patient, making his word law. Here medicine becomes an instrument at the service of radical subjectivism. The patient is a consumer, the doctor a provider of services who must put his scientific expertise at the service of the patient's subjective wishes and desires.[15] This is the ideology of self-realisation in which my health and my body, that is, my physical well-being, have become an instrument within my life projects, to be used and transformed at wish and will, instead of it being a physical aspect of myself that is 'mine' in a manner that goes beyond my full control.[16]

How can we avoid both radical opposite movements? First of all, it is important to acknowledge that providing room for the physician as a scientific expert and for the success of the medical treatment on the one hand, and leaving room for the preferences and wishes of the patient on the other hand, are *both* fundamental aspects of the medical experience. Nevertheless, when interpreted with radical unilateralism, both aspects threaten to get bogged down in an authoritarian attitude of the physician on the one hand, and a demanding or consumerist attitude of the patient on the other.

[15] For a closer view on the problems of medicine on demand, see a.o. L. BOUCK-AERT, 'Gezondheid en solidariteit: oude en nieuwe veronderstellingen' [Health and Solidarity, Old and New Presuppositions] in J. HALLET, J. HERMESSE & D. SAUER (eds.), *Solidariteit, gezondheid, ethiek* [Solidarity, Health, Ethics] Leuven-Apeldoorn, Garant, 1994, pp. 49-56; K. DEMYTTENAERE, 'Medisch begeleide voortplanting: spel zonder grenzen?' [Assisted Reproduction: Game without Limits?] in B. RAYMAEKERS, A. VAN DE PUTTE & G. VAN RIEL, (eds.), *Moeten, mogen, kunnen: ethiek en wetenschap* [To Have, To May, To Can: Ethics and Science], Leuven, Universitaire Pers, pp. 148-158.

[16] See also: R. BERNET, 'Doen zonder denken en denken zonder doen' [Action without Thought, Thought without Action] in H. DE DIJN, *Ingrijpen in het leven. Fundamentele vragen over bio-ethiek*, Leuven, Universitaire Pers, 1988, pp. 73-84.

Nevertheless, however good the intentions of a doctor may be, imposing a treatment without the patient's consent is commonly interpreted as a violation of human rights and the patient's dignity. Moreover, however important it is to acknowledge the patient as a human being whose wishes must be taken into account, the physician is not a puppet whose services are at one's beck and call for the achievement of personal happiness.

With the development of the informed consent doctrine, medicine has distanced itself from the naturalistic and functionalistic interpretation of medicine. In its original sense the principle of autonomy, in the form of giving one's free and informed consent, refers to the fact that medicine is a *relational* practice. Medical decision-making is a process of *sharing* the decision between patient and physician. Both parties are indispensable on the road to a prudent and proper decision: on the one hand the physician functions as the expert with his experience and scientific knowledge where diagnosis of the patient's state of health and prognosis of various treatments are concerned, and on the other hand the patient knows his particular life goals and values, which can be influenced differently by various treatments.

The medical experience as a shared event between patient and physician reflects a solidarity model (as I demonstrate in Figure 3 below). This model stresses the mutual alliance between doctor and patient and as such, it abandons objectivistic, naturalistic and functionalistic paternalism as well as the subjectivistic autonomy interpretation.[17]

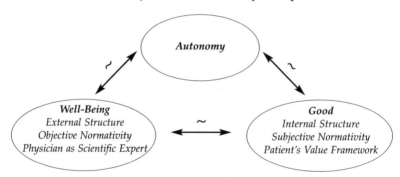

Figure 3: The Solidarity model

Respect for medicine as an objective science concerning human biological functioning is not put aside in this view. On the contrary, since

[17] This model approaches the argument of 'beneficence in trust' elaborated by E.D. PELLEGRINO and D.C. THOMASMA in their work *For the Patient's Good: the Restoration of Beneficence in Health Care*, New York, Oxford University Press, 1987.

it is a physical science the goal of medicine is still improving the patient's health, understood as physical well-being. As such, and understood from the perspective of the threefold model I illustrated before, medical intervention and care aim at protecting and promoting a patient's autonomy in the best possible way. In this case, and it is important to mention it again, autonomy is interpreted as biological or functional autonomy, that is as physical independence, which has an objective normativity with respect to the medical task. It refers to the objective normative standard of physical well-being, independent from individual preferences or values.

Additionally, the subjective normativity of autonomy includes respect for the patient's personal balancing of pros and cons of a series of alternative treatments, according to his personal values, convictions, preferences and emotions. In other words, according to his individual interpretation of the good life.[18]

According to this view, respect for the patient's autonomy in medical decisions implies a necessary combination of autonomy as both objective and subjective normativity. A human being does not fully coincide with his physical functionality: as a person he transcends biological objectivity but at the same time he continues to be connected to it. This means that a person's *physical well-being* is necessarily a determining factor of a person's life projects, that is, of his views of *the good life*, his life plans, wishes, preferences and desires, and the decisions he accordingly makes in shaping his life. Inversely, his view on the *good life* will inevitably determine the way he relates to his physical *well-being*, in this case the decisions he makes with respect to medical treatment.

3. Autonomy, Dependence and Care

Let us now consider the third and final issue. When it is not or no longer possible for medical intervention to provide a reasonable level

---

[18] In order to have a plausible preference theory on the good life, there must be room for 'laundering' personal preferences. Discussion of this issue and extensive bibliography in R.E GOODIN, 'Laundering Preferences' in ID., *Utilitarianism as a Public Philosophy*, Cambridge, Cambridge University Press, 1995, pp. 132-148. On the possible conflict between preferences and values related to the concept of the good life, see H.G. FRANKFURT, 'Freedom of the Will and the Concept of the Person' in ID., *The Importance of What We Care About. Philosophical Essays*, Cambridge, Cambridge University Press, 1988, pp. 11-25.

of autonomy for the sick or disabled person, autonomy being under-stood as self-determination *both in thought and action*, possessing both a subjective and an objective normativity, we have to take care of this person in the best possible way so as to make his situation of depen-dence the best of a bad situation.

Against the background of human finiteness and the inevitable sit-uation of psychological or physical dependence, which presents itself to most people at certain times in their lives — that is in cases of childhood, illness, handicap and old age — dependence has an *onto-logical* status. As argued extensively by Eva Kittay and Martha Nuss-baum, dependence is an essential characteristic of human existence.[19]

Although autonomy or independence can also be seen as an essen-tial characteristic of human existence, just as Heidegger's famous concept of 'Geworfenheit' includes the duty of personal 'Entwurf', an important difference between autonomy and dependence never-theless remains. Autonomy is universally seen as a normative value, worthy of protection and promotion. In spite of human finiteness, dependence, on the other hand, is *not* seen as a goal worthy of pro-tection and promotion. On the contrary, one tries to promote, retain, and realise autonomy and agency as long as possible in spite of the limits of human existence; and this is by all means the first task of medicine. Accordingly, medical intervention and medical care have an important emancipating function.

Nevertheless, one has to beware of a blind glorification of the idea of care. To help and care is not universally and unconditionally vir-tuous, however good the intentions may be. This goes against a pos-sible interpretation of an ethics of care, which supports the view that the *more* we are prepared to help each other and the *more* concerned

---

[19] E.F. KITTAY, *Love's Labor. Essays on Women, Equality, and Dependency*, New York, Routledge, 1999; ID., 'Can Contractualism Justify State-Supported Long-Term Care Policies? Or "I'd Rather Be Some Mother's Child,"' in WORLD HEALTH ORGANIZATION, *Ethical Choices in Long-Term Care. What Does Justice Require?*, Geneva, World Health Organization, 2002, pp. 77-83; M.C. NUSSBAUM, 'The Future of Feminist Liberalism,' in *Proceedings and Addresses of the American Philosophical Association* (2000)74, pp. 47-79; ID. 'Disabled Lives: Who Cares?' in *The New York Review of Books* 48(2001)1, pp. 34-37; ID., 'Long-Term Care and Social Justice. A Challenge to Conventional Ideas of the Social Contract,' in WORLD HEALTH ORGANIZATION, *Ethical Choices in Long-Term Care. What Does Justice Require?*, Geneva, World Health Organization, 2002, pp. 31-65; ID., 'Beyond the Social Contract: Toward Global Justice,' in G.B. PETERSON (ed.), *The Tanner Lectures on Human Values*, vol. 24, Salt Lake City, University of Utah Press, 2004, pp. 413-507.

we are with care, the better human beings we are.[20] As taken into account by care ethicists as Joan Tronto for example, care is ambiguous, as it includes the risk of being too caring.[21] This can be clarified again by the threefold connection between autonomy, physical well-being and the good life.

As a person one is inevitably connected to one's physicality, one's health condition, which I have defined as physical *well-being*. This connection to one's physicality co-determines a person's identity. This identity however, is not solely determined by how one looks, how one *functions* mentally and physically, whether or not one is healthy, whether or not one needs help, but *also* by one's projects, life plans and actions, for example, interests in travelling, hiking, writing et cetera. In other words, by the life projects one pursues and fulfils as an individual which are an exteriorisation of one's individual conception of the *good life*. The importance that is commonly attached to the fact that one can actually carry out one's life-plans, that one can determine and actually do freely what one believes is important and meaningful, illustrates the role of *autonomy* in this matter.

Contrary to the conventional view, as illustrated in figure 1, I believe that autonomy as self-rule and self-governance should not be taken as an *independent* and *isolated* value. Whatever one autonomously chooses to do, it is not a random choice but always a response to what emerges as *meaningful* and to what one appreciates in life. For example we respond to what our friends and family have already done or not done with their lives. The normativity of autonomy is illustrated by the fact that parents hope that their children will 'do their own thing', 'stand on their own two feet', and shape their own lives. This wish has both an *objective* component, reflected by the child's *physical* well-being, and a *subjective* component, incorporated in the child's pursuit of the *good life*.

In a sudden or slowly increasing situation of dependence, for example due to accident or ageing, the patient is challenged to confront their dependence, possibly reviewing their earlier life projects and to organise their life in relation to this dependence. It is possible that the patient reacts with grief, and emotions like shame or aggression, and that he

---

[20] Philosophical critique on this view can also be found in M. SLOTE, 'The Justice of Caring' in *Social Philosophy and Policy* 15(1998), pp. 171-195 and in A. BURMS, 'Helping and Appreciating' in S. GRIFFIOEN (ed.), *What Right does Ethics Have? Public Policy in a Pluralistic Culture*, Amsterdam: VU University Press, 1990, pp. 67-77.

[21] J. TRONTO, *Moral Boundaries. A Political Argument for an Ethic of Care*, New York, Routledge, 1993.

demonstrates behaviour such as increased self-care and avoidance of further risk, in order to find a way to cope with the situation. The same goes for people with a severe congenital handicap.

In coping with this situation of dependence one tries to establish autonomy in the best possible way, no matter how, but in trying to make the best of this bad situation a 'too caring' care overshoots this goal. Patronising, controlling and authoritative care causes resentment and too much help can lead to aggression. The feeling of intrusion on one's privacy (as was the case for Ramon Sanpedro) not only refers to the fact that the care-giver comes too close to one's personal space and activities in a physical way, for example in washing or changing, I believe it also relates to the fact that a 'too caring' care hinders one's subjective and personal creativity in coping with one's physical situation in the light of one's conception of the good life, a creativity which is nevertheless still there.

Too much help may look like a substitute for subjective creativity, a negation of autonomy *in* dependence. As Nick Fox puts it "Sometimes, one's attempts to give (however well-intentioned) do not enable, but disable".[22] This arouses conflict because one wants to *do* things *oneself*, albeit with some help. One refuses to get stuck in a unilateral situation of dependence.

Theories on the logic of the gift indicate the problem of a unilateral gift to which one can respond only with gratitude. Such gifts corner the receiver within his inferiority and as such arouse frustration. To give, receive and be able to return are rooted in the fundamental human desire for social acknowledgement. To offer a person the possibility of reciprocity implies the acknowledgement of the other as an autonomous person, as a subject endowed with activity and creativity.[23]

Applied to care, it is often the case that in a situation of dependence the subjective creativity is not gone: the patient often redevelops himself through an active and performative process. With the necessary help and care, the person *himself* wants to rediscover his autonomy and what that means in his particular situation. When care is given in full recognition of the other as an autonomous and

---

[22] In: N. Fox, 'Postmodern Perspectives on Care: the Vigil and the Gift' in *Critical Social Policy* 15(1995), pp. 107-125, p. 122.

[23] A. Vandevelde, 'Towards a Conceptual Map of Gift Practices' in Id. (ed.), *Gifts and Interests*, Leuven, Peeters, 2000, pp. 1-20; A. Burms, 'Helping and Appreciating' 1990.

creative subject *in* dependence, the unilateral gift turns into the gift of freedom and possibility.

In this context Nick Fox stresses the importance of the "appropriate lightness of care."[24] For care to enable a person to be autonomous in dependence, the caring activity must emphasise generosity instead of control, individual identifications (like, "This is Adrian, June, my father, our neighbour") instead of demeaning, patronising, and totalising reductions (which appear in labels such as "the handicapped," "the sick," "the dependent," "the one that needs to be taken care of"). Caring must make room for a person's individual choices and for the diversity of people in forming and pursuing their concept of the good life. This is opposed to the view which interprets the ill individual as a mere deviation of the objectively, naturalistically and functionalistically defined health norm. An 'appropriate lightness of care' offers possibilities and room for activity and subjective creativity:

> "The objective of care in this perspective has to do with *becoming* and *possibilities* [...]. It is a process, which offers *promise*, rather than fulfilling it, offers *possibility* in place of certainty, *multiplicity* in place of repetition, *difference* in place of identity. It is the *gift* which expects no recognition."[25]

The previously analysed solidarity model in which the *objectivity* of physical well-being and the *subjective* creativity of the personal implementation of the *good life* come together, in other words, in which *autonomy* is understood as a joint venture of objective and subjective normativity, is probably the best possible way to approach the art of giving care without humiliating.

References

AMENÁBAR, A. (dir.), *Mar Adentro* (*The Sea Inside*), Time Warner, Fine Line, 2004.

BEAUCHAMP, T.L. & CHILDRESS, J.F. *The Principles of Biomedical Ethics*, New York, Oxford University Press, 2001.

BERNET, R., 'Doen zonder denken en denken zonder doen' [Action without Thought, Thought without Action] in H. DE DIJN (ed.), *Ingrijpen*

---

[24] See: N. FOX, 'Postmodernism and Health' in A. PETERSEN & C. WADDELL (eds.), *Health Matters: A Sociology of Illness, Prevention and Care*, Buckingham, Open University Press, 1998, pp. 9-22, p. 20.

[25] In: N. FOX, *Ibid.*, p. 21.

in het leven. Fundamentele vragen over bio-ethiek [Intervening in Life. Fundamental Questions on Bioethics], Leuven, Universitaire Pers, 1988, pp. 73-84.

BOORSE, C., 'On the Distinction between Health and Disease' in *Philosophy and Public Affairs* 5(1975), pp. 49-68.

BOUCKAERT, L., 'Gezondheid en solidariteit: oude en nieuwe veronderstellingen' [Health and Solidarity, Old and New Presuppositions] in J. HALLET, J. HERMESSE & D. SAUER (eds.), *Solidariteit, gezondheid, ethiek* [Solidarity, Health, Ethics], Leuven-Apeldoorn, Garant, 1994, pp. 49-56.

BROCK, D., 'Quality of Life Measures in Health Care and Medical Ethics' in M.C. NUSSBAUM & A. SEN (eds.), *The Quality of Life*, Oxford, Clarendon Press, 1993, pp. 95-132.

BURMS, A., 'Helping and Appreciating' in S. GRIFFIOEN (ed.), *What Right does Ethics Have? Public Policy in a Pluralistic Culture*, Amsterdam: VU University Press, 1990, pp. 67-77.

CAPLAN, A.L. (et al.), *Concepts of Health and Disease: Interdisciplinary Perspectives*, Reading, Addison-Wesley, 1981.

DE DIJN, H., *De herontdekking van de ziel. Voor een volwaardige kwaliteitszorg* [The Rediscovery of the Soul. Towards a Full Quality Care.], Nijmegen, Valkhof Pers, 1999.

DELEUZE, G. & GUATTARI, F., *Anti-Oedipus: Capitalism and Schizophrenia*, London, Athlone, 1984.

DEMYTTENAERE, K., 'Medisch begeleide voortplanting: spel zonder grenzen?' [Assisted Reproduction: Game without Limits?] in B. RAYMAEKERS, A. VAN DE PUTTE & G. VAN RIEL, (eds.), *Moeten, mogen, kunnen: ethiek en wetenschap* [To Have, To May, To Can: Ethics and Science], Leuven, Universitaire Pers, 2001, pp. 148-158.

DIERICKX, K. *Genetisch gezond? Ethische en sociale aspecten van genetische tests en screenings* [Genetically Healthy? Ethical and Social Aspects of Genetic Tests and Screenings], Antwerpen, Intersentia, 1999.

FOX, N., 'Postmodern Perspectives on Care: the Vigil and the Gift' in *Critical Social Policy* 15(1995), pp. 107-125.

FOX, N., 'Postmodernism and Health' in A. PETERSEN & C. WADDELL (eds.), *Health Matters: A Sociology of Illness, Prevention and Care*, Buckingham, Open University Press, 1998, pp. 9-22.

FRANKFURT, H.G., 'Freedom of the Will and the Concept of the Person' in ID., *The Importance of What We Care About. Philosophical Essays*, Cambridge, Cambridge University Press, 1988, pp. 11-25.

GOODIN, R.E., 'Laundering Preferences' in ID., *Utilitarianism as a Public Philosophy*, Cambridge, Cambridge University Press, 1995, pp. 132-148.

HÖFFE, O., *Immanuel Kant*, München, Beck, 2000.

KANT, I., *Kritik der praktischen Vernunft*, Hamburg, Meiner, 1990.

KASS, L., *Towards a More Natural Science*, New York, Free Press, 1985.

KITTAY, E.F., 'Can Contractualism Justify State-Supported Long-Term Care Policies? Or "I'd Rather Be Some Mother's Child,"' in WORLD HEALTH ORGANIZATION, *Ethical Choices in Long-Term Care. What Does Justice Require?*, Geneva, World Health Organization, 2002, pp. 77-83.

KITTAY, E.F., *Love's Labor. Essays on Women, Equality, and Dependency*, New York, Routledge, 1999

MILL, J.S., *On Liberty*, s.l., Wordsworth, 1859 (ed. 1996).

NUSSBAUM, M.C., 'Beyond the Social Contract: Toward Global Justice,' in G.B. PETERSON (ed.), *The Tanner Lectures on Human Values*, vol. 24, Salt Lake City, University of Utah Press, 2004, pp. 413-507.

NUSSBAUM, M.C., 'Disabled Lives: Who Cares?' in *The New York Review of Books* 48(2001)1, pp. 34-37.

NUSSBAUM, M.C., 'Long-Term Care and Social Justice. A Challenge to Conventional Ideas of the Social Contract,' in WORLD HEALTH ORGANIZATION, *Ethical Choices in Long-Term Care. What Does Justice Require?*, Geneva, World Health Organization, 2002, pp. 31-65.

NUSSBAUM, M.C., 'The Future of Feminist Liberalism,' in *Proceedings and Addresses of the American Philosophical Association* (2000)74, pp. 47-79.

PARFIT, D., *Reasons and Persons*, Oxford, Clarendon Press, 1984.

PELLEGRINO, E.D. & THOMASMA, D.C. *For the Patient's Good: the Restoration of Beneficence in Health Care*, New York, Oxford University Press, 1987.

SLOTE, M., 'The Justice of Caring', in *Social Philosophy and Policy* 15(1998), pp. 171-195

TAYLOR, C., *Sources of the Self. The Making of the Modern Identity*, Cambridge, Harvard University Press, 1989.

TRONTO, J., *Moral Boundaries. A Political Argument for an Ethic of Care*, New York, Routledge, 1993.

VANDEVELDE, A., 'Towards a Conceptual Map of Gift Practices' in ID. (ed.), *Gifts and Interests*, Leuven, Peeters, 2000, pp. 1-20.

4. INFORMED CONSENT AND THE GROUNDS OF AUTONOMY

David Archard

The obtaining of informed consent to any medical intervention or for participation in any medical research is a core bioethical precept. The obtaining of consent is said by the principal defenders of the requirement to be a 'specification' of the principle of respect for individual autonomy. It is as much a specification of this principle as the requirements upon doctors to "tell the truth" and "protect confidential information".[1] Consent is viewed as the 'central conceptual tool in the protection and expression of personal autonomy' — not simply within medicine but in structuring conventions that govern all our interpersonal and political relationships.[2] In turn the principle of respect for autonomy is regarded as one of the four governing principles of ethical practice, the other three being justice, beneficence and non-maleficence.

In recent years there has been extensive criticism of the requirement of informed consent and of the importance assumed by the principle of autonomy. It has been suggested that autonomy has acquired a position of pre-eminence enjoying priority over the other three principles. Such priority is an unwarranted 'triumph' inasmuch as it represents the influence of atomic individualism over the claims of social membership and relatedness. A medical culture regulated by the principle of beneficence is essentially paternalistic, a principle of justice recognises our duties to one another as fellow citizens, whilst a principle of patient autonomy acknowledges that each person is entitled by and on her own to determine what shall happen to her.

---

[1] T.L. BEAUCHAMP & J.F. CHILDRESS, *Principles of Biomedical Ethics*, 4th edition, Oxford, Oxford University Press, 1994, p. 127.

[2] S. CLARKE, 'Informed Consent in Medicine in Comparison with Consent in Other Areas of Human Activity' in *Southern Journal of Philosophy* 39(2001), p. 172.

The requirement of informed consent has come under attack from both social scientists and philosophers. Social scientists believe that a full and proper acknowledgement of social processes — the circumstances under which people make choices, the pressures to which they are subject when doing so, the forms of manipulation and influence to which vulnerable individuals are subjected to by figures of medical authority — reveal the abstract principle of informed consent to be an 'empty' and formalistic requirement.[3] For their part philosophers are dubious whether patients can be sufficiently informed or deliberatively rational when deciding about their own medical future, and will allege that respect is not owed simply to expressions of personal choice, the mere assertions of preference.[4]

The interesting question underlying such varied criticisms, though not often spelled out, is what is supposed to make consent the essential tool in the protection of individual autonomy. Why is it thought that obtaining consent from patients and medical research subjects is indispensably necessary to ensuring that they are respected as autonomous beings? This contribution is devoted to trying to answer this question.

I

Tom Beauchamp and James Childress note that there have, historically, been two sources for the insistence upon the necessity of obtaining informed consent. The first was that consent functioned to ensure that the harms done to and injustices suffered by individuals were minimised.[5] Contemporary bioethical thinking is deeply influenced by the codes of medical practice that emerged in explicit reaction to the excesses of the Second World War. Thus the Nuremberg Code of Ethics, itself a product of the Nuremberg War Crimes Trials of 1945, sought to specify and fix the rights of human subjects in research experiments. At the forefront of the minds of those who devised this code were the abhorrent practices of German physicians, nurses and

---

[3] See, for instance, O. CORRIGAN, 'Empty Ethics: The Problem with Informed Consent' in *Sociology of Health and Illness* 25(2003), pp. 768-792.

[4] See, for instance, Onora O'Neill's helpfully brief summary of views she defends elsewhere at length: O. ONEILL, 'Some Limits of Informed Consent' in *Journal of Medical Ethics* 29(2003), pp. 4-7.

[5] T.L. BEAUCHAMP & J.F. CHILDRESS, *Principles of Biomedical Ethics*, p. 142.

scientists who engaged in experimental research upon prisoners without their knowledge or willing agreement. The Nuremberg Code led to the Declarations of Helsinki which, in successive forms, have been drafted by the World Health Organisation.[6]

Imposing a duty upon medical personnel to consult with their patients or subjects, and giving these latter persons a right to refuse or accede to any proposal is a way of ensuring that they do not suffer any ills, or serious risks thereof, of which they are not fully aware or which they are not prepared to undergo. The historical context for the first formulation of a principle of informed consent makes perfect sense of its prophylactic role in safeguarding the interests of otherwise vulnerable individuals. However, as Beauchamp and Childress note, the second justification for the principle — and the one that has been advanced in recent years — has been the protection of autonomous choice.

Autonomous choice, and its protection by means of consent, has a general significance within modern Western liberal societies. It is central to our normative understanding of the relations in which we as individuals stand to one another, and to the authorisation of any instruments of legitimate control over us. Thus, for instance, the dominant paradigm of liberal sexual autonomy is one in which what matters — indeed all that matters — is that sane, mature adults give willing permission to one another for their behaviour. Whatever is freely consented to is permissible, and whatever is not consented to is utterly impermissible. Rape is the gravest sexual wrong, and all sexual practices, however 'perverted', are allowable so long as consensual.[7]

Again, an influential account of the source of the authority of the state over us is that we, as individuals, have given our consent to its creation. This account has canonical formulations in the writings of John Locke and Thomas Hobbes, and continues to exercise enormous influence over contemporary political philosophical thinking on the problem of political obligation. This is so despite the many, oft-repeated expressions of scepticism about the possibility of citizens giving any kind of consent — express, tacit or implicit — to the state.[8]

[6] For a good brief history of the subject, see B.P. DENNIS, 'The Origin and Nature of Informed Consent: Experiences Among Vulnerable Groups' in *Journal of Professional Nursing* 15(1999), pp. 281-287.

[7] For my own analysis of this paradigm of sexual morality, see D. ARCHARD, *Sexual Consent*, Oxford, Westview Press, 1998.

[8] The best critical review of the ideal of political consent is A.J. SIMMONS, *Moral Principles and Political Obligations*, Princeton, Princeton University Press, 1981.

Grant that the ideal of autonomy is a central ideal, and also allow that we think of consent as itself key to the protection of autonomy. Why, nevertheless, should we continue to believe that informed consent to *any* medical intervention is such an important requirement? Let me take as an instance of a relatively trivial or minor medical intervention the obtaining of information by means of a simple mouth swab. This is painless, relatively cheap, takes very little time, and involves the most inconsequential intrusion upon the person.

Let me, further, point out what enormous good might and often can be done as a result of securing and processing the information the swab makes possible. Obviously a swab allows for a DNA profiling of the person from whom it is taken. Such a profile might assist in the identification of a criminal, and the prevention, thereby, of future serious crimes. The victims of those possible crimes are spared. The swab might assist in the identification of the person carrying a lethal, and highly infectious, disease. His isolation or treatment spares the lives and health of those who would otherwise contract the disease. The processing of the swab might simply contribute to the expansion of our knowledge of the human genome, and, as a result, to the benefits such knowledge brings in its wake. None of these suggested benefits are fanciful; nor are they anything but substantial. Why, then, should we think that no swab should be taken without the informed consent of the individual, and why should we think that this requirement rests ultimately upon the central principle of respect for autonomy?

II

Autonomy is self-rule. The capacity of individuals to govern themselves, to determine the direction of their lives, obviously varies, and some individuals are more autonomous than others. Nevertheless insofar as we can agree on a threshold of autonomous decision-taking the principle of autonomy directs that we should respect the choices of others so long as they are, in the minimally specified degree, autonomous. A decision is autonomous if it is sufficiently informed, sufficiently voluntary, and sufficiently rational. There are significant and persisting differences of philosophical opinion as to what counts as sufficient in all three respects. However I shall set such disputes to one side, because the critical question under consideration is why we should respect the choices of others inasmuch as they are autonomous however that is specified.

The two obvious — and certainly the most influential — philosophical sources of warrant for the ideal of autonomy are Kant and Mill. Kant is an unpromising source for the ideal insofar as what for him is owed respect is not simply the free choices of others but the exercise of practical reason in conformity with the moral law. If contemporary Kantians, such as Onora O'Neill, are deeply sceptical of the principle of informed consent it is precisely because they believe that there is a huge difference between respecting rational autonomy and respecting the preferences of individuals. The latter may be the individuals' own and may be freely expressed. Yet they need not be autonomous in the way that Kant intended and which he explicitly tied to the moral law.

> Contemporary accounts of autonomy have lost touch with their Kantian origins, in which the links between autonomy and respect for persons are well argued; most reduce autonomy to some form of individual independence, and show little about its ethical importance.[9]

If Kant is an unpromising source for the contemporary ideal of personal autonomy what then of John Stuart Mill?

The Mill of *On Liberty* famously defends the liberty of individuals "in the maturity of their faculties" to make choices so long as their chosen actions do not adversely affect the interests of others. Mill never uses the language of autonomy but his celebration of 'individuality' and 'spontaneity' resonates with contemporary defences of the ideal. Notoriously, however, Mill explicitly sets his defence of individual liberty within the context of his utilitarianism. His appeal is not to abstract right, but to the principle of utility insofar as it is "utility in the largest sense, grounded on the permanent interests of man as a progressive being".[10] However he does not make it clear whether liberty — autonomy for our purposes — has an intrinsic or an instrumental justification. Is it that autonomy is valuable inasmuch as autonomous choices are productive to the overall good of the person, because, for instance, individuals are probably best placed to know what is good for them, or because, it is best on

---

[9] O. O'NEILL, 'Some Limits of Informed Consent', p. 5.
[10] J.S. MILL, *On Liberty*, ed. G. HIMMELFARB, Harmondsworth, Penguin, 1974, p. 70.

balance, to assume that they are since the costs of acting on a contrary assumption are negative? Or is that choosing one's own life is
itself an ineliminable and essential element of what it is to lead a
good life?

What does seem clear — and it is relevant to our discussion — is
that for Mill, and his contemporary defenders, autonomy is valuable
when set within the leading of lives, not when making occasional isolated decisions of little or no significance. Autonomy is to be evaluated in the context of major life-affecting choices and across life-
times; we do not value autonomy — or we do not value it to any
significant degree — merely when it allows us a one-off choice from
the restaurant menu of a main course. Autonomy is global not occur-
rent. It is concerned with "a whole way of living one's life and can
only be assessed over extended periods of a person's life".[11]

Once again then it is hard to see why the right of consenting or
refusing a mouth swab is to be protected as part of what it is to
respect individual autonomy. For how is that a short-lived intrusion
into a mouth cavity, even if uninvited and unwelcome, subverts the
ability of its victim to lead her life as she chooses? How is her autonomy denied by this unconsented intervention? However this particular example prompts a number of thoughts that might confuse the
matter. Moreover it is all too easy to conflate the value of autonomy
with that of other important personal interests. Two confusions in
particular need to be addressed.

III

The first confusion arises from the natural thought that what is
wrong with obtaining the swab without consent is that it violates not
autonomy but *privacy*. What the investigator secures access to is the
properly protected domain of another's privacy. Privacy is a distinct
ideal to that of autonomy. This is so even though many who claim to
defend the ideal of autonomy do so in terms that are recognisably
those of Millian liberty. For instance, the Irish Law Reform Commission's Report on Privacy defends privacy as providing "vital space

---

[11] G. DWORKIN, *The Theory and Practice of Autonomy*, Cambridge, Cambridge University Press, 1988, pp. 15-16.

for personal growth and development and for the exercise of freedom".[12]

Still, it might be thought that both privacy and autonomy share common ground and that this has to do with the ability of any person to lead her life by her own lights. On the favoured definition of privacy it is restricted access to a protected sphere of personal information. The right to privacy is a "right to limit public access to oneself and to information about oneself".[13] "A person has privacy to the extent that others have limited access to information about him, limited access to the intimacies of his life, or limited access to his thoughts or his body".[14] "[P]ersonal privacy is a condition of inaccessibility of the person, his mental states, or information about the person to the senses or surveillance devices of others."[15]

On this account what is objectionable about the unconsented swab is not so much its being done as such but rather the processing and use of the information thereby gained. What seems wrong is that others get to know about the victim of the swab what they would otherwise not know. Of course even this does not quite seem to get at what is wrong with the swab. For, as viewers of many TV police and hospital dramas will know, exactly the same DNA information can be obtained from traces innocently left on coffee cups, cigarette butts, toothbrushes, and hairbrushes.

Moreover, just as we can distinguish between the act of taking the swab and the information gained in consequence so we can further distinguish between the mere possession of such information and its use. Note then that someone can consent to the taking of the swab but not to its being processed, or can consent to the processing of the swab but not to the general dissemination of the information gained. What seems objectionable — and what then does seem to allow privacy to share ground with autonomy in terms of an ability to lead one's own life — is the employment of personal knowledge in ways

---

[12] THE LAW REFORM COMMISSION (IRELAND), *Report on Privacy: Surveillance and Interception of Communication*, Dublin, The Law Reform Commission, 1998, p. 3.

[13] A.D. MOORE, 'Privacy: Its Meaning and Value' in *American Philosophical Quarterly* 40(2003), p. 218.

[14] F. SCHOEMAN, 'Privacy: Philosophical Dimensions' in F. SCHOEMAN (ed.), *Philosophical Dimensions of Privacy: An Anthology*, Cambridge, Cambridge University Press, 1984, p. 3.

[15] A.L. ALLEN, *Uneasy Access, Privacy for Women in a Free Society*, Totowa, NJ, Rowman & Littlefield, 1988, p. 15.

that are constricting of personal choice. Personal information of this kind can be used by the state to determine who shall be prosecuted, detained, interned or quarantined. Personal information of this kind can be used by private individuals who come into its possession in order to coerce, manipulate, control, and blackmail the other.

Expressed in these ways the wrongness of gaining access to personal information is more naturally spoken of as a breach of confidentiality. Indeed many writers would prefer that we speak in these terms than by resort to a problematic category of privacy. What the taker of the swab does wrong — if she makes use without the other's consent of the personal information she acquires — is to break a confidence. She has no right to exploit information she could only have gained by refusing to honour an agreement, explicit or implicit, with the other person.

A breach of confidentiality is a refusal to respect the other's choices; one person comes to know something other than by being willingly told or being allowed to find out. A breach of confidentiality is in this sense a display of disrespect for another's autonomy, her freely expressed wishes. Yet confidentiality is not the same thing as privacy. Moreover the breaking of a confidence would be wrong for being the defiance of another's wishes, even if it had no significant impact on the ability of the other to lead her life. Imagine, then, that I disclose to the public what I have been told in confidence about another's long dead relative. This knowledge cannot seriously undermine the capacity of the other to conduct her life as she chooses. Yet I do a serious wrong in revealing what I was entrusted to keep secret.

In sum, if the taking of the swab is wrong for being a violation of privacy or a breach of confidence it is wrong ultimately for reasons other than its being a disrespecting of autonomy. Or rather although autonomy is disrespected in the straightforward sense that another's wishes are not honoured what is done does not vitiate the ability of the other to lead her life as she chooses, and this, as argued, is what gives autonomy its value.

A second confusion does not arise from this particular example but can be discerned in the following general line of reasoning that concerns the relationship between consent, information, and autonomy. The more information relevant to the making of a choice that can be obtained the more autonomous the subsequent choice can be. Obviously at the threshold of autonomy someone can lack sufficient salient information to make an autonomous decision; similarly one can possess just enough information to make a decision that is sufficiently autonomous to merit protection. Since information enhances autonomy in this way obtaining informed consent plays a part in promoting and enlarging autonomy.

However being under an obligation to obtain informed consent does not mean, nor does it entail, being under an obligation to provide the information that would ensure that the consent is informed. Someone under an obligation to obtain informed consent is required not to do without consent that for which the consent is needed — the operation or the experiment, for instance. The doctor wishing to perform the operation or the researcher wishing to conduct the experiment has a reason to give the subject relevant information. He has such a reason insofar as he thinks that the provision of such information will lead the other to give her informed consent to the operation or experiment. Yet he can discharge the obligation to proceed only if informed consent is given even when he is not himself the source of the relevant information. If Dr. Smith proceeds with an operation on Susan to which she has consented he acts permissibly. He does so even if the details of the operation — its nature, risks, likely consequences, feasible alternatives — have been provided by Dr. Jones. It is enough that Susan's consent to Dr. Smith's actions is informed; it is not required that she is informed *by Dr. Smith* about his actions.

So, the obligation to obtain consent is not an obligation to inform and hence to do that which would enhance autonomy in that way. Obtaining consent may amount to a respecting of the other's wishes, but it is not of itself nor does it necessitate the enhancement of autonomy by supplying information. Of course it is arguable that a doctor or experimenter ought to tell the truth when questioned about his proposal; or that he ought to help another make her choices by providing the relevant information. However he is not obligated to do so simply because he must obtain her consent.

IV

An understanding of why the unconsented mouth swab amounts to a violation of the principle of respect for autonomy cannot then be found by thinking either in terms of privacy or of the relationship between information, consent and autonomy. Yet sticking a swab in someone's mouth without their permission seems evidently wrong and it would still seem to be wrong even if the swab was immediately destroyed and no personal information were obtained nor could be used. It would be wrong even if done when the subject was asleep, unaware of the imposition, and felt no discomfort.

At this point the ideal of *self-ownership* suggests itself. The thought is that each person is, as Mill expressed it, 'sovereign over his own body'. I own my embodied self and you trespass upon this personal space when, without my permission, you take a swab, stick a needle into me, or otherwise physically interfere with me. You violate my self in this respect even if the trespass is minor and harmless in its consequences. After all I trespass upon your land — and wrong you — even if I only take one step into your territory and do no damage to the ground.

The idea of self-ownership can be traced to John Locke who notably used it as the premise in a celebrated argument, via labour, for private ownership: "every Man has a *Property* in his own *Person*. This no Body has any Right to but himself."[16] This intellectual provenance is interesting if only because Locke is often characterised as a father of modern philosophical liberalism. Yet Kant, already cited as a source for the ideal of autonomy and himself a clear influence upon modern philosophical liberals, rejected the very idea of the person as owning herself. The person is, for Kant, improperly conceived as an object which can be possessed: "Man cannot dispose over himself because he is not a thing; he is not his own property; to say that he is would be self-contradictory; for insofar as he is a person he is a Subject in whom the ownership of things can be vested, and if he were his own property, he would be a thing over which he could have ownership. But a person cannot be a property and so cannot be a thing which can be owned, for it is impossible to be a person and a thing, the proprietor and the property."[17]

The idea of self-ownership is embraced by contemporary left libertarians such as Hillel Steiner and Peter Vallentyne.[18] Yet it is important to disengage the ideal of self-ownership from the intellectual

[16] J. LOCKE, *Two Treatises of Government*, ed. P. LASLETT, Cambridge, Cambridge University Press, 1963, II, section 27.

[17] I. KANT, *Lectures on Ethics*, trans. L. INFIELD, Indianapolis, Hackett, 1963, p. 211.

[18] See P. VALLENTYNE & H. STEINER (eds.), *Left Libertarianism and its Critics: The Contemporary Debate*, Houndmills, Palgrave, 2000.

architecture constructed by those who employ it as a foundational stone. Thus no scheme of distributive justice should be taken as endorsed in consequence of affirming the basic ideal. At its simplest the ideal is the affirmation of a reflexive relationship in which the embodied self stands to itself. Moreover it enjoys the most basic of relations to consent. "To say that A enjoys self-ownership is just to say that A owns A: 'self', here, signifies a reflexive relation".[19] And to say that A is self-owning is just to say that things cannot be done to A without A's consent.

The question that now arises is as to how we should understand the ideal of self-ownership in relation to that of autonomy classically conceived as self-rule. Is sovereignty over one's body an implication or consequence of a more primitive ideal of self-determination? The judgement in Nathanson v. Kline affirms as much: "Anglo-American law starts with the premise of thorough-going self-determination. It follows that each man is considered to be master of his own body, and he may, if he be of sound mind, expressly prohibit the performance of lifesaving surgery".[20] Or is self-ownership an ideal distinct from but as irreducibly basic as that of autonomy?

It is important to get this clear because some discussions appear to run the ideals together or leave it unclear which ideal is being appealed to. Consider the claim by Beauchamp and Childress that "[a]n informed consent is an *autonomous authorization* by individuals of a medical intervention or of involvement in research".[21] On one reading 'autonomous' characterises the source of the authorisation. An individual is authorised to consent to a medical intervention insofar as he is an autonomous person whose choices in this matter should be respected. On another reading 'autonomous' characterises the manner in which the authorisation is given, namely freely, knowingly and rationally. Yet the source of the authorisation is an open matter. It could be the idea of the individual as possessed of autonomy that merits protection. Or it could be the individual as a self-owning agent; intrusions into whose space demand his permission.

---

[19] G.A. COHEN, *Self-Ownership, Freedom and Equality*, Cambridge, Cambridge University Press, 1995, p. 211.

[20] Nathanson v. Kline, 186 Kan. 393 at 406, quoted in G. DWORKIN, *The Theory and Practice of Autonomy*, p. 101.

[21] T.L. BEAUCHAMP & J.F. CHILDRESS, *Principles of Biomedical Ethics*, p. 143; italics in original.

V

How then might we think of the relationship between autonomy or self-determination and self-ownership? Gerald Dworkin and Joel Feinberg both think of interferences with my body as violations of my autonomy albeit for different reasons. However I am not persuaded that we can think of bodily self-ownership as following from self-rule. Let me say something about the reasoning of each.

For Dworkin self-rule grounds bodily ownership because my body is 'me' in some very significant way. One's body is, he says, "irreplaceable and inescapable". Since my body *is me*, "failure to respect my wishes concerning my body is a particularly insulting denial of autonomy".[22] It does indeed seem true that to treat my body against my will in certain ways — by physically assaulting me, raping me, mutilating me — is to show disrespect for my choices in an especially serious manner. No violation of my person can be felt so profoundly damaging and hurtful as one which breaks the skin, cuts into my flesh or invades my body. A gross interference with another's body can be a gross violation of her autonomy. Yet it need not be; nor need a gross violation of another's autonomy involve a gross bodily interference.

In the first place, the significance for Dworkin of my body being me is that my wishes in respect of it are directly, and especially, insulting to me. Yet whilst a person's body is indeed irreplaceable and inescapable (though not all of its parts are to the same extent) the value of a body to its owner may vary. Someone who attaches a particular significance to something other than his own person ('It means more to me even than my own life') will feel his autonomy more insulted by having his wishes regarding it not respected than he would be by a serious assault on his person. A religious ascetic might care little for his physical self and much more for objects of his religious devotion.

In the second place the body is not an indivisible, unitary and bounded entity any interference with which possesses the same significance. Its various parts and elements have different significance for us. We shed skin, hair, nails; we expel bodily fluids. It is surely false that all losses from my body which should, on this account, be losses of some part of 'me' have the same meaning. There is a huge

---

[22] G. DWORKIN, *The Theory and Practice of Autonomy*, p. 113.

difference between my taking while you sleep your kidney and my cutting your hair or nails.

Thirdly what gives autonomy its value, as we have seen, is its role in the directing of one's life across extended periods of time. A gross interference with my body could limit my ability to make significant life choices. Consider the unwilled amputation of a major limb; yet some gross bodily interferences will have the effect of enhancing or preserving choice. Consider the removal of a major tumour that was restricting or would in the future seriously restrict movement: the operation to remove the tumour would enhance autonomy. This is true even if the operation was not consented to, as would be the case if the tumour was discovered in the course of routine minor exploratory surgery and removed before the patient could agree to its removal. Moreover it seems to me that the patient's autonomy would be enhanced even if he not only could not give his consent but — inferring from prior expressed wishes and views — would not have consented to the tumour's removal.

By contrast the grossest interferences with autonomy can be managed without any violation of bodily space. Consider the issuing of a credible threat to inflict death or serious injury upon a woman's infant child should she not comply with the terms of the threat. Such a threat would be coercive and as such significantly limits the autonomy of the mother. Yet it does not involve any interference, actual or possible, with the body of the mother, nor does it involve actual interference with any body.

I am my body it is true. But it does not follow that my autonomy is a simple and direct function of my bodily integrity. Violations of autonomy are not the greater the grosser the interferences with my body. If violations of body space are to be evaluated as more or less serious it must be by reference to a standard derived not from the ideal of self-rule but from that of bodily self-ownership.

Joel Feinberg argues for a direct relationship between self-rule and bodily self-ownership in the following manner. Personal choice, he says, is about "where and how to move my body through public space".[23] Feinberg thinks as he does because he envisages self-rule as sovereignty exercised over a personal domain that extends beyond the will to one's body and even to one's "breathing space". Moreover he thinks that this sovereignty should be untrammelled: "one is

---

[23] J. FEINBERG, *Harm to Self*, Oxford, Oxford University Press, 1986, p. 54.

entitled to absolute control of whatever is within one's domain however trivial it may be".[24]

On Feinberg's account the same wrong is done to an owner however significant the trespass and however serious the harm done to the property by the trespasser. This may be plausible if one is thinking in terms of ownership. However it does not sit easily, as Feinberg himself recognises, with the ideal of autonomy when this is cashed out in terms of a "right to decide how one is to live one's life, in particular how to make the critical life-decisions".[25] Moreover an absolute ideal of bodily sovereignty does not seem to play the right kind of role in justifying the exercise of personal choice.

Crucial here is the asymmetry between doing things with one's body and having things done to one's body. In the first place the analogy with sovereign nation-states that Feinberg himself invokes breaks down. It is certainly true that on a simple Westphalian model a nation, a group of individuals, or even an isolated individual does wrong in crossing without permission the boundaries of a sovereign state. The wrong is that of invasion. Yet it certainly does not follow that nation-states, sovereign over their own territory, have a right to move through international space. Indeed for them to do so would precisely amount to the wrong of invading other nation-states. Yet Feinberg seems to think that a right not to have one's own bodily space invaded is essentially paired with a right to move one's body through public space.

In the second place talk of a right to move one's body through public space surely misdescribes or underspecifies what is essentially involved in the exercise of autonomy. Denying someone the right of private, silent religious contemplation is not best viewed as the violation of a right of the devotee to move his body through public space. Many important life-choices are not about what to do with one's own body but what to think or believe, and — one of Feinberg's own examples — what virtues to cultivate. The contents of such choices are not essentially or significantly about bodily movements.

Once again it is a mistake to think that ownership or control of one's body is a simple consequent or expression of a right of choosing one's life. It would be better to think that one has a right to make

---

[24] *Ibid.*, p. 55.
[25] *Ibid.*, pp. 54-55.

critical life choices — autonomy — and that one also has a distinct putative right to control what is done to one's body — self-owner-ship. This brings us back once again to the example of the mouth swab. If this requires informed consent it cannot be because this is demanded by respect for personal autonomy. It may be because one should respect the right of the owner of the mouth to refuse a tres-pass upon this particular orifice. But understood in these terms it is just as unclear that a serious wrong is done in obtaining the mouth swab as it would be if we were to think in terms of significant life-choices being denied.

I conclude that the ideal of autonomy — specified within the bioethical context as the principle of informed consent — is not per-spicuously or securely grounded. Furthermore I conclude that many of the putative wrongs done in not securing informed consent within the medical domain are not best understood as violations of auton-omy but rather as breaches of the principle of self-ownership, an ideal quite distinct from that of autonomy.

References

ALLEN, A.L., *Uneasy Access, Privacy for Women in a Free Society*, Totowa, NJ, Rowman & Littlefield, 1988.

ARCHARD, D., *Sexual Consent*, Oxford, Westview Press, 1998.

BEAUCHAMP T.L. & J.F. CHILDRESS, *Principles of Biomedical Ethics*, 4th edi-tion, Oxford, Oxford University Press, 1994.

CLARKE, S., 'Informed Consent in Medicine in Comparison with Consent in Other Areas of Human Activity' in *Southern Journal of Philosophy* 39(2001), pp. 169-188.

COHEN, G.A., *Self-Ownership, Freedom and Equality*, Cambridge, Cam-bridge University Press, 1995.

CORRIGAN, O., 'Empty Ethics: The Problem with Informed Consent' in *Sociology of Health and Illness* 25(2003), pp. 768-792.

DENNIS, B.P., 'The Origin and Nature of Informed Consent: Experiences Among Vulnerable Groups' in *Journal of Professional Nursing* 15(1999), pp. 281-287.

DWORKIN, G., *The Theory and Practice of Autonomy*, Cambridge, Cam-bridge University Press, 1988.

FEINBERG, J., *Harm to Self*, Oxford, Oxford University Press, 1986.

KANT, I., *Lectures on Ethics*, trans. L. INFIELD, Indianapolis, Hackett, 1963.

LOCKE, J., *Two Treatises of Government*, ed. P. LASLETT, Cambridge, Cam-bridge University Press, 1963.

MILL, J.S., *On Liberty*, ed. G. HIMMELFARB, Harmondsworth, Penguin, 1974.

MOORE, A.D., 'Privacy: Its Meaning and Value' in *American Philosophical Quarterly* 40(2003), pp. 215-227.

ONEILL, O., 'Some Limits of Informed Consent' in *Journal of Medical Ethics* 29(2003), pp. 4-7.

SCHOEMAN, F., 'Privacy: Philosophical Dimensions' in F. SCHOEMAN (ed.), *Philosophical Dimensions of Privacy: An Anthology*, Cambridge, Cambridge University Press, 1984.

SIMMONS, A.J., *Moral Principles and Political Obligations*, Princeton, Princeton University Press, 1981.

THE LAW REFORM COMMISSION (IRELAND), *Report on Privacy: Surveillance and Interception of Communication*, Dublin, The Law Reform Commission, 1998.

VALLENTYNE P. & H. STEINER (eds.), *Left Libertarianism and its Critics: The Contemporary Debate*, Houndmills, Palgrave, 2000.

5. IS AUTONOMY RELEVANT TO PSYCHIATRIC ETHICS?

Eric Matthews

The more I reflect on the concepts of paternalism and autonomy — especially but not only in the context of psychiatry — the more confused and dissatisfied I become. The principle of respect for patient autonomy is supposed to be an expression of the value of the individual patient: but, since autonomy can be respected only if it exists, and since mental illness is held by many to consist of a loss of autonomy, that seems to imply that individuals with mental illness have no value, no human dignity to be respected. That seems counterintuitive, and suggests that the opposition of paternalism and autonomy may not be the best framework for thinking about the ethics of the doctor-patient relationship, at least in psychiatry and perhaps in medicine more generally. In this contribution, I want to explore this issue, with particular reference to psychiatry, although in order to do so, I first need to think in a wider context about the rejection of medical paternalism and the rise in importance of respect for patient autonomy.

I

Traditional medical ethics, as expressed for instance in the Hippocratic Oath, rested on an essentially hierarchical conception of the doctor-patient relationship. It was the doctor's duty to do what was best for the patient, regardless of what the patient him- or herself thought of the proposed treatment. "Doctor knew best", and it was the patient's duty to "obey doctor's orders". This was not only a duty, but was in the patient's own self-interest: it was assumed that the patient would, if rational, agree with the doctor's conception of what was a desirable outcome, and so with the doctor's medically informed view of the best way to achieve that outcome. This was a *power* relationship: the doctor's superior knowledge gave him (it was virtually always a "him") the right to make treatment-decisions on the patient's behalf, and thus excluded the patient from any active role in making those decisions. Just as a tree-surgeon can make a tree 'better' without any concern with what the tree feels, so a medical doctor can, on this view, make a patient better without reference to the patient's feelings about what is done to him or her.

This was 'paternalism' because it was like the traditional conception of the relationship of a parent, especially a father, to his children. Fathers had the authority to make decisions on behalf of their children, at least up to the age at which they became adults, and the children simply had to obey without question. In the same way, doctors were authority-figures, in a quasi-parental relationship with their patients. All this was called into question by the modern liberal critique of traditional views of human relationships. Two elements of modern liberalism in particular were important: the dissolution of a general consensus about what was good in human life, and the growth of a belief in the equal worth of all human beings. The first was taken to mean that patients and doctors would not necessarily agree about what was a desirable outcome of medical treatment; and the second meant that the patient's view of what was desirable was of equal value to the doctor's — the idea of the doctor as an authority-figure was undermined. The analogy of the doctor-patient relationship to that between father and child ('paternalism') came to be seen as insulting to adult patients: especially since the relationship of parents to children was itself reformulated in liberal thought (a point I shall return to later). The decision of a normal adult human being about what was to happen to his or her own body must have final authority.

Yet this cannot follow simply from the fact that it is the patient's life and well-being which are at stake in medicine. If doctor knows best, not only about medical technicalities, but also about what is in the patient's best interests, then it would be sensible to allow the doctor to have the final say about treatment. It is only if the patient's conception of what is best for him or her is of equal value to that of the doctor that it might reasonably be held that the patient should be the ultimate decision-maker. It is here that the notion of "autonomy" enters. As Beauchamp and Childress say, the term is borrowed from political thought.[1] In the equally liberal notion of the sovereign

---

[1] T.L. BEAUCHAMP & J.F. CHILDRESS, *Principles of Biomedical Ethics*, 5th edition, New York, Oxford University Press, 2001, pp. 57-58.

nation-state, each state is supposed to be 'autonomous', or self-governing, making its own laws to regulate its own national life, in accordance with its own values, and without interference by any other state or body. Each state is assumed to be the best judge of what is best for itself, and the judgements of one state may validly differ from those of others.

How can these political conceptions be transferred to individual human beings? What makes each individual, in the characteristically liberal term, 'sovereign' over his or her own destiny? One answer to this is proposed by Kant, in what I take to be the first philosophical use of the term 'autonomy' in relation to individuals. Kant specifically compares reason to the legislature. Reason is supposed to evaluate possible maxims of conduct to determine whether they are such as could be laws of a society of rational beings (whether they could be 'universalised'). Individuals are autonomous, for Kant, to the extent that they regulate their own conduct, from a moral point of view, by such universalisable maxims, just because they can see, by the exercise of their own pure practical reason, that they are universalisable. Individuals do their duty in so far as they act in accordance with what Reason shows to be their duty, and regardless of their individual wishes or desires.

Thus, for Kant, autonomy deserves respect because it is an essential part of human rationality: the decisions of the individual are valued, not just because they are the decisions of that individual, but because they are based on the human capacity to act from reason alone, disregarding the promptings of personal desire or impulse, or even considerations of the individual's own self-interest. Rational decisions in the relevant sense are, on Kant's conception, those which are based on pure moral principle, not those based on what has been called 'instrumental' or 'means-end' rationality — calculations of the best means to achieve a given end, where the end cannot itself have a rational foundation. This makes 'autonomy' in the Kantian sense very different from the 'patient autonomy' which is supposed to be respected in modern medical ethics.[2] In the *Principles of Biomedical Ethics*, the autonomy of the patient is supposed to consist in basing treatment decisions on his or her own conceptions of value, of what is 'good for me', or in the patient's long-term self-interest, as he or she sees it, regardless of whether that view of the good would be

---

[2] See also E. MATTHEWS, 'Autonomy and the Psychiatric Patient' in *Journal of Applied Philosophy* 17(2000), p. 1.

generally regarded as rational. But if so, then the moral grounds for insisting that autonomy should be respected must also be different from those proposed by Kant. Kant was concerned with *moral* decision-making: the modern conception is concerned rather with *non-moral* good, with what is good in the sense of what an individual may prefer.

Another possible foundation for a principle of respect for patient autonomy in this sense might be found in J.S. Mill's dictum that "the only purpose for which power can be rightfully exercised over any member of a civilised community, against his will, is to prevent harm to others ... over himself, over his own body and mind, the individual is sovereign".[3] Individuals, for Mill, must be allowed to make their own decisions about how they should live, even if their decisions do not meet with general approval as sensible, provided only that the consequences of those decisions do not cause harm to others. If they do cause harm, then they are morally objectionable by Mill's Utilitarian criteria: so the individual's choice of a way of life is not, it seems, motivated by *moral* considerations, but only by the individual's personal preferences. If we see the doctor-patient relationship as one in which the doctor at least potentially exercises power over the patient, for instance in making treatment decisions, then Mill's principle would entail that such an exercise of power can be 'rightful' only when it is intended to prevent harm to others. If there is no question of harm to others, then the patient must make the ultimate decision, in accordance with his or her own preferences. It is the patient's body and mind which these decisions concern, and the patient is 'sovereign' over them.

Is this a mere dogmatic assertion on Mill's part, or does he have some supporting argument for his principle? The best place to look for such an argument is in what he says in the same essay (*On Liberty*) about 'experiments in living'. Because human beings are imperfect, he argues, it is impossible for anyone to be certain about what is the best life. Therefore, we ought to allow individuals to experiment with their own conceptions of the good life for them, even if such individual conceptions may not conform to generally accepted conventions. Allowing people to cultivate their own individuality in this way is, he argues, the only way which "produces, or can produce,

---

[3] J.S. MILL, *On Liberty and Other Essays*, ed. J. GRAY, Oxford, Oxford University Press (World Classics), 1998, p. 14.

well developed human beings".[4] This is therefore a kind of Utilitarian argument: the overall social consequences of allowing people to experiment in this way will be beneficial, producing diversity and fully developed human beings.

Mill does not actually use the word 'autonomy', but what he says about experiments in living and their value does fit in with one use of that term, which does refer to something we value in modern liberal society. Liberal parents seek to encourage in their children the growth of 'autonomy' in the sense of the capacity to make their own decisions about life, based on conceptions of value which they have developed for themselves, by their own thinking. Babies and small children, being at the beginning of this process of development, clearly have not yet formulated their own values, so that decisions about their lives have to be made for them by adults (normally their parents or guardians) who care for them and have their long-term well-being at heart. Thus, a child may be unwilling to go to the dentist because of a fear of short-term pain. Caring parents will take account of such fears and seek to allay them: but, if they genuinely care for the child's long-term welfare, they will make the decision on the child's behalf to go to the dentist, to avoid the possibility of much greater pain and distress in the future. This is literal 'paternalism', and most people would not find it morally objectionable, at least in the case of very small children (on the contrary, it would be morally irresponsible for parents to fail to make such decisions on the child's behalf).

With increasing years, however, such 'paternalism' ceases, in a liberal view, to be morally acceptable. According to modern conceptions of the duties of a parent, there is an obligation to make possible and encourage their child's development to autonomous adulthood, to becoming an independent human being. The child should be increasingly encouraged to formulate her own views about what is desirable in life, and to make her own decisions. In the modern jargon, she must 'take ownership of' the values which govern her decisions. 'Paternalism' (whether on the part of those who are literally parents or of those others who care for someone, such as doctors) is morally objectionable when it consists of treating an adult as a child — treating someone who is acting on values which she has formulated for herself as if she were not capable of doing so. 'Autonomy' in this

---

[4] *Ibid.*, p. 71.

sense is a feature of normal adulthood, so that respecting it is part of our general respect for all adults as equals.

It does not follow, however, that every decision made by an adult is worthy of respect, since experience shows that not every decision is based on thought-through values. Mill himself does not regard all choices of ways of life as respectable 'experiments in living'. For instance, he regards choices made by those adults who are mentally incapacitated and so need the care of others as not worthy of respect.[5] Why not? Because respectable experiments in living must be rationally defensible. Although Mill, as stated earlier, holds that human reason is imperfect, he still insists that we should exercise our reasoning faculties as far as they will take us. We must do the best that human reason is capable of: if we do so, "we have neglected nothing which could give truth a chance of reaching us".[6] The clear implication of this is that there *is* a truth about the best way of living, even if imperfect human beings can never be certain that they have reached it. The lack of certainty, *not* the impossibility in principle of objective values, is the justification for allowing a variety of experiments in living. Nevertheless, these experiments need to be grounded in the exercise of reason, even in its imperfect form: acceptable experiments must rest on "a standing invitation to the whole world to prove them unfounded". They must be shown to be based on values which others can see at least to be rationally intelligible, as possible objective values, even if they do not themselves share those values.

Mill's discussion applies most obviously to those situations in which people act on thought-out values, but in which it is held to be impossible to be certain about which of these values is in some objective sense 'correct'. Two typically liberal institutions exemplify this situation: the market and political democracy. In a market, consumers make choices between the goods and services offered by suppliers. The consumers have reasons for their preferences, but different consumers may have different reasons for their different preferences, and it is held to be impossible to say which of these preferences is objectively correct. For instance, in the housing market, one person might want to buy a house in the country with a large garden, another to buy a flat in the middle of town. Either preference can be

[5] *Ibid.*, p. 14.
[6] *Ibid.*, p. 26.

defended by rational arguments, but it seems impossible to say that one preference is more rational than the other: so no one is entitled to impose one choice of house by the exercise of power. The individual is sovereign in such choices. Similarly, in a political democracy, one set of voters may value social and economic equality more highly than liberty, whereas another set may value liberty over equality. Again, the proponents of each ideology can offer arguments in favour of their own position, but no such arguments can conclusively *prove* the truth of that position. Liberals therefore conclude that the authoritarian imposition of libertarianism or egalitarianism (or any other ideology), as in a totalitarian society, is wrong: the ideology which prevails at any given time must be the one preferred by the majority of those affected. Liberal democracy therefore again presupposes the sovereignty of the individual over his or her own life — the autonomy of the individual.

Insistence on respect for the autonomy of the individual as a central principle of medical ethics implies that the doctor-patient relationship is in important respects like that between suppliers and consumers in a market economy, or between government and citizens in a liberal democracy. Is it? There seem to be some morally significant differences between the two situations. First, and perhaps most important, it does seem that there are certain principles of value in health care which are 'objective', at least in the sense that any rational person would agree to them, indeed failing to agree to them would in itself be a mark of irrationality. We could give several examples of such principles which are relevant to medical decision making. For instance, that continued life without great suffering or distress (or where the cause of suffering or distress has been removed by medical treatment) and in a conscious state (or where consciousness can be restored by medical treatment) is preferable to death. Or that medication which may relieve suffering or distress should be accepted, provided that the suffering or distress caused by the medication itself does not outweigh that which it relieves. A final example, particularly relevant to mental illness, would be that a life which is reasonably under one's own control is preferable to one which is not. These seem to me to be principles which any rational person, in so far as she is rational, would accept as obvious. Of course, they are formulated in very general terms, and there might be reasonable disagreement about their application in particular cases. For instance, we might differ about how long life should be prolonged by invasive medical treatment, even if it does relieve suffering or distress, or about the point at which the distress caused by medication out-weighs that which it relieves, or about the degree of control which we want over our own lives. Moreover it is not irrational (though it is not usual) to think that other values might be higher than those of health and control of one's life, for example, achieving spiritual depth or eternal blessedness. Yet someone who thinks in these terms would presumably not be involved in medical decision making, and those who are so involved would not seek medical help unless they accepted at least the general principles as self-evident.

Another difference between the doctor-patient relationship and that between suppliers and consumers in a market is that we see the doctor as someone more than a mere technician, providing ser-vices which are regarded as good simply because the "consumers" (patients) prefer them. We seek medical help when we are in distress and want the medical profession to help us out of that distress. The doctor in turn has always been regarded as under a moral obligation (unlike the commercial supplier of consumer goods) to consider the patient's well-being as more important than his or her own: to do his or her best (medically speaking) for the patient, even if he or she does not personally benefit from the transaction. Doctors respect the human dignity of patients by doing their best for their health.

How does this affect the principle of respect for patient autonomy? First of all it seems to entail that respect for patients' human dignity does not necessarily mean accepting patients as the ultimate decision makers in medicine, since clearly not every decision which a patient may make conforms to one of the rational principles listed earlier. Patients even with bodily illnesses are, after all, often in a highly vul-nerable condition — in the emotional turmoil which results from great pain or weakness, or in a barely conscious state, and thus are unable to function as rationally as they normally would. To picture them as consumers in the market-place, making cool decisions about what they prefer, is absurd and demeaning to them. In the most extreme case, the patient is unconscious and so totally unable to make any kind of decision at all. Our existing codes of medical ethics allow doctors in such cases to make decisions on the patient's behalf, at least in pursuing emergency life-saving measures.

On the other hand, patients, at least those who are adult or well on the way to adulthood, are, as fellow human beings, the equals of doc-tors, and so have a right to be consulted about the treatment they are

to receive, as far as that is possible. There is no ethical room for paternalism, if that means doctors simply deciding as they see fit, without
consultation of any kind with patients. Ideally, consultation should
take the form of an actual dialogue with the patient, in which the
patient's possible reasons for wishing a different treatment from that
proposed by the doctor are explored and taken with full seriousness.
It may well be that the patient is not being as irrational as the doctor
may initially have thought. For instance, the patient may accept the
objective principles outlined above in their general terms, but may
have a different interpretation of how they apply to his or her own
case. An example might be a different, but perfectly reasonable, conception of the value of achieving a relatively short period of continued life by means of highly invasive treatment like chemotherapy.
Since this is a reasonable opinion to hold, it ought to be respected by
the doctor: this is a case where the patient, as an adult, ought to be
allowed to "take ownership" of decisions about his or her own life,
because the doctor's differing views about treatment have no claim
to be regarded as more rational.

This is the ideal: but of course in the real world things are not often
like this. There are practical difficulties, such as the sheer lack of time
and opportunity for such an exploratory dialogue. These difficulties
can to some extent be overcome, or at least alleviated, by discovering
what the patient's own views would have been, if there had been
time for a full exploration: this can be done, for instance, by reference
to advance directives, where they exist and are relevant, or to
appointed proxy decision-makers, or to family members or close
friends. These indirect methods are always dangerous, but it may be
that they are the best we can hope for in such circumstances.

However there is also another problem, in some ways more serious. Even if there is time for a serious exploration of the patient's
views about treatment, it might still turn out that by any standard
they are without reasonable foundation, especially with the most vulnerable patients. The difference between doctor and patient may consist, not in their respective interpretations of how to apply general
principles to the particular case, but in their understanding of what
those principles themselves imply. Suppose, for instance, the doctor
judges (rightly, from the point of view of medical science) that a
particular patient requires high doses of powerful antibiotics, delivered intravenously over a substantial period of time, if a grave risk
of serious blood infection is to be avoided. For practical reasons, the

intravenous injections can be given only in hospital. The patient, however, is so depressed at the prospect of a further long stay in hospital that she wants to refuse the injections. She is in denial about the risk of infection, and cannot be persuaded to see otherwise however much the doctor seeks to argue with her, and however sensitively the doctor explores her own view of the position. What should doctors do in this situation? Legally, they may well be required to get patient consent before doing anything, but I am concerned with issues of ethics, rather than law. The ethical question is, how can they best respect their patient's human dignity? It seems to me that the answer here is, by acting as it is rational to do for the patient's benefit, not by accepting the patient's own decision at the time. If the patient herself would come to regard this as the best decision when she is in a state more open to rational thought, and if acting autonomously is acting in a rationally defensible way, then this could even be seen as respecting the patient's autonomy: but this is not how this principle is often interpreted.

This is not advocating medical paternalism as traditionally conceived. It is not suggested that the doctor is in a superior position to make decisions because of his or her professional status. Doctors and patients are equals. The doctor is no more likely to be rational about the patient's best interests than the patient: indeed, in some ways the doctor's very professional training may incline him or her to certain judgements which need not necessarily be more reasonable, for example, that it is always better to prolong life even by means of highly invasive treatment which may actually diminish the quality of the remaining life. The argument is rather that the patient's real decision may be apparent only after exploratory dialogue, investigation of advance directives and the like. Also, more controversially, there may be ethical justification for acting contrary to the patient's currently expressed wishes if, after thorough exploration of the kind suggested, those wishes seem irrational to any normal person, including the patient herself when she is in a calmer mood.

II

In general medicine, then, I have argued that respect for the patient's human dignity requires doctors above all to act in the patient's best interest, preferably, but not necessarily, with the patient's consent, and where all practicable steps have been taken to get the patient's rational consent. How does this apply to the special case of psychiatric medicine? In much of psychiatric treatment, of course, the ethics of treatment decisions is not all that special. Patients with less severe mental disorders, such as the phobias, are no more likely than patients with bodily illnesses to fail to recognise that they have a problem which needs professional help, and that they would be well-advised to follow the advice of those professional helpers if they wish to be rid of the problem. If their initial responses seem irrational, they are just as likely to be open to changing their minds (or perhaps to persuading the psychiatrist to change hers) as a result of the kind of exploration of their reasons which has been described.

The more difficult problems arise with more serious psychiatric conditions, such as schizophrenia, major depression and dementia. Here the very nature of the illness itself in part consists in loss of autonomy, to such an extent that it may seem a mere waste of time and effort to engage in exploratory dialogue with the patient. Patients are likely to deny that they have a psychiatric problem at all, and so that their behaviour, its affects and so on, need treatment of any kind. They may therefore refuse the hospitalisation and medication which the psychiatrist sees as essential if they are to be helped. They may neglect their personal hygiene, or engage in other forms of self-harm, including attempts at suicide, and may resent efforts to prevent them harming themselves in these ways. Their behaviour may harm others around them in unacceptable ways. This is why, in all jurisdictions that I know of, there is legislation making it possible in certain circumstances to confine psychiatric patients in hospital and to treat them against their will, for their own benefit and/or for the protection of others.

In line with the earlier argument, therefore, it might seem that the ethically right thing to do is for the psychiatrist in such cases to make treatment decisions on the patient's behalf, even if the patient at the time explicitly refuses such treatment, provided that the choice is made on rational grounds which patients themselves could recognise as such when they were in a more 'normal' state of mind. In those rare cases in which they exist, psychiatric living wills could be used as evidence that this would indeed have been the patient's wish if they were capable of rational decision-making. Others close to the patient could also be consulted for their views of what the patient would have wanted. Though in the end, the psychiatrist would have to rely on his or her own judgement — once again, a dangerous course of action, but perhaps unavoidable. To this extent, the answer to the question posed in the title of this chapter would be that autonomy was not relevant in psychiatric ethics when dealing with such cases, at least if "respect for patient autonomy" is taken to mean acceptance of the wishes regarding treatment which the patient expresses at the time. However, taken in a broader sense, of respect for the patient's *rationally considered* wishes, respect for autonomy is as relevant in psychiatric ethics as in any other field of medicine.

Yet whether or not a patient lacks autonomy at the time is anyway irrelevant from the point of view of respecting his or her human dignity: respect is shown by doing the best for the patient, and in this context that means above all endeavouring to restore the patient's autonomy. The psychiatrist, like all medical professionals, is under an ethical obligation to do what is best for the patient, as the patient would see it if rational, and it is in fulfilling that obligation that the psychiatrist best shows respect for the patient as an equal fellow human being. Helping patients to return as far as possible to the same kind and degree of control over their own lives as most people have, ought to be a primary aim of psychiatric treatment.

This does seem to be the only conclusion to be drawn from the earlier arguments. However, there are some complicating factors to be considered which imply that psychiatrists should not be too quick to assume that their patients lack autonomy at the time when they are presented. First of all, the difficulties of psychiatric diagnosis are well known. Behaviour, beliefs or affects which may at first glance seem to be symptomatic of mental illness may on closer examination come to be seen as intelligible, and in their own way reasonable, responses to real situations. What may look like paranoid delusions of persecution may turn out, for instance, to be perfectly reasonable beliefs based on evidence of real persecution. Or again, suppose an old lady experiences lapses of memory and begins to behave in ways which her family find hard to cope with. As a result, she is diagnosed with dementia and removed against her will to a psychiatric hospital. There she becomes increasingly obstreperous, destroying ornaments in her room, verbally abusing staff and other patients, and making phone calls to her relatives, demanding to be taken away from "this horrible place". Her carers conclude that these are further symptoms of her dementia, and decide to put her in a secure ward, where this behaviour can be better controlled, for what they see as her own good, and perhaps to give her medication for the same purpose.

However might not another interpretation of her behaviour be possible? Her difficult behaviour at home might not be entirely the result of her dementia, but in part the kind of thing which might be expected from someone of her temperament, faced with the prospect of old age and the sense that her dreams for her own life would never be fulfilled. What looked like lapses of memory might in fact be only partially a result of deterioration in the relevant parts of her brain: to some extent, they may be a kind of stratagem on her part to draw the attention of her family to her problems. The obstreperous behaviour in the hospital might be an understandable human reaction to the feeling that her control of her own life had been forcibly removed from her. Exploring these possibilities with her might not be a waste of time. Psychiatrists have to be on their guard (more so than specialists in bodily medicine) against the tendency, resulting from their professional training, to interpret all sorts of deviant human behaviour as symptoms of mental disorder. If this lady's behaviour can reasonably be understood in this way, then she would still have problems (as would her family). These problems would probably still require psychiatric treatment, but a greater understanding of how she felt might have a bearing on *how* this treatment was applied — even to the way in which doctors and nurses spoke to her about the treatment. Above all, exploring the patient's inner reactions in this way involves seeing the patient as a fully equal fellow human being, and not simply as a 'case', to be helped from the outside.

A second sort of complication is this; even if a person is genuinely suffering from a psychiatric disorder, so that some of her beliefs and behaviour are genuinely irrational, it does not follow that she is incapable of making rational treatment decisions. Someone who suffers from a delusion, for example hearing the voice of God inside her head, instructing her to do certain things, may still be capable of weighing the costs and benefits of proposed treatments in a rational way: is it for example worth putting up with the possibly unpleasant side-effects of some medication for the sake of the relief which the drugs may give from the consequences of her condition? Of course, some delusions might have a direct bearing on the rationality of such calculations: for instance, she might believe that her doctors are trying to poison her with the drugs they are offering. Yet not all delusions or other psychotic symptoms are of that kind. Once again, it is not an entire waste of time to explore the patient's reasons for wanting to refuse treatment.

Again, some things which look to the psychiatrist like delusions may play a useful role in the patient's life and may not be delusions in any real sense, so the patient may have understandable grounds for not wanting treatment for them. The psychiatrist, having had a scientific training, may well, for instance, regard some of a patient's religious beliefs, especially if they are not part of any mainstream religious creed in the psychiatrist's culture, as necessarily irrational and in need of treatment. Though they may give coherence and meaning to the patient's life, and if so it is not irrational to wish to hold on to them, and to resist any suggestion that they are symptoms of a mental disorder and need to be treated by psychiatric methods.

It is, of course, a well-known feature of at least some of the more severe forms of mental illness that the patient denies that she is ill at all. This is indeed one of the most difficult features of psychiatric practice (though denial that one is ill is not entirely unknown in somatic medicine). Clearly, if one is convinced one is not ill, then it is not irrational to refuse therapy, especially if one knows that it has undesirable side-effects. The psychiatrist, on the other hand, may well be equally convinced that the patient is ill, and that the denial is itself part of the illness, so that there is a professional obligation to treat that illness by the very methods that the patient refuses. Caution is required, however. Psychiatrists, as stated earlier, have a tendency, derived from their professional training, to see mental disorder in any kind of deviant behaviour. It shows respect for the patient to devote at least some time to dialogue aimed at discovering whether this tendency is justified in this case before proceeding to impose treatment on the patient against her wishes. Yet if such dialogue takes place, and no evidence is found that the patient's thoughts or behaviour are simply unusual, rather than disordered, then the argument of this chapter would imply that respect for the patient's humanity positively *requires* the psychiatrist to act against that patient's presently expressed wishes.

In one particular case, I would want to argue that it is always justified to act in what some might regard as a 'paternalistic' fashion. One of the characteristic features of clinical depression is 'suicidal ideation' — that is, constant thoughts of taking one's own life and a standing inclination to put those thoughts into practice. Those who are not depressed may also contemplate suicide as a solution to their problems, but may be open to persuasion that it is not a real solution. Genuinely depressed people will not be open to such persuasion, and can be prevented from committing suicide only by removing the opportunities for taking their own lives. The question is, is it ethical to act in this preventive way, contrary to the person's own sincerely expressed wishes? I would argue that it must be. The psychiatrist's professional obligation is to help patients and, if possible, to find genuine solutions to their problems. But ending one's life cannot be a genuine solution to any problems in one's life: it is cutting through the Gordian knot rather than untying it. Indeed, it clearly removes all possibility of finding a genuine solution to one's problems. This is especially true of the kinds of problems which require psychiatric help. Yet even in cases where there may be some doubt about the psychiatric diagnosis, and so some possibility that there may be grounds which some might regard as rational for the desire to end it all, there is an obligation on anyone in the relevant position to make every possible effort to prevent suicide. To simply acquiesce in a person's desire to take her own life, when one has some possibility of preventing her from killing herself, may be to respect her autonomy, but it is also a failure to treat her life as of equal value to one's own, and so is lacking in a deeper respect for her worth as a human being.

III

So what is the final answer to the question posed in this chapter? The conclusion of the discussion could be expressed in what may seem to be a bland way: "sometimes autonomy is relevant to psychiatric ethics, sometimes it isn't". This is not as bland an answer as it sounds: it is a way of saying that the ethics of the doctor-patient relationship, especially (but not only) in psychiatric cases is more complex than it is often depicted as being. The conflict between medical paternalism and respect for patient autonomy provides a framework for thinking about this relationship which is not exactly wrong, but may be misleading. Traditional medical paternalism did indeed reflect a hierarchical society in which deference was owed to those of higher status, and that kind of society is incompatible with the liberal conceptions which we (or most of us) nowadays accept. In modern liberal thinking, deference is out of place, at least in secular relationships like that between a doctor and a patient. Doctors must resist any temptation to think of themselves as superior to their patients: medicine exists for the *patients'* sakes, and so any superior knowledge which the doctor has in virtue of her professional training must not be a mark of status, but a means by which she can serve the patients' interests.

All this could be expressed as a principle of respect for patients and their human worth. Yet to use the term 'autonomy' in the statement of this principle is misleading, because it focuses attention too much on one aspect of respect for patients, as if doctors had to respect their patients in so far as, and only in so far as, they are rational decision makers. For much of the time, most patients can make perfectly rational decisions about treatment or non-treatment, as judged by the kind of rational principles referred to earlier in the paper. Because they are rational, they will probably coincide with those which doctors make, so that there will be no problem about asserting patient autonomy *against* paternalistic doctors. An adult human being *ought* to take ownership of decisions about her own life in this way, and doctors ought to encourage adults to do so. But what makes these decisions worthy of respect is mainly that they do have a rational basis. Sometimes, when patients are in a particularly vulnerable state, because of the frailty of their condition, their first response to a proposed course of treatment may be far from rational. Then respect for the patient's humanity requires a doctor, if at all possible, to explore the decision further with the patient, including dealing sensitively with the feelings which may have led to this irrational decision. The patient's humanity is not contained only in her powers of rational thought, important though these are, but in feelings which may take some time and effort to elicit, but which are, once elicited, intelligible to most other human beings. If intelligible, they make sense of the patient's seemingly bizarre initial decision and certainly need to be taken into account if the patient is to be persuaded to make a more rational choice of treatment. Alternatively, the doctor may come to see that the patient's initial choice was more rational than it seemed at the time: accepting that possibility is part of respecting the patient's equal humanity.

But what if there is no time in practice for this kind of exploration, or if, after all the exploration of reasons and feelings, the patient still wants to stick with a decision which a more detached view can see to be contrary to that patient's own best interests? In that case, it seems to me that the respect for the patient's humanity which ethics requires implies that the doctor should act in what is the patient's best interests, even if the patient herself does not presently see things that way (remember that I am talking about ethical, rather than legal, requirements, which may be completely different). This is not 'paternalism' if the doctor acts in what the patient herself would see to be in her own best interests, if only she were in a more rational frame of mind, which indeed she may well be later when feeling better and come to see as having been in her best interests. Of course, the doctor needs to support her judgement of what the patient would think in any way possible, for example by advance directives, relatives opinions, or judgements of the patient's appointed proxy.

In the case of psychiatric disorders, there are more complications. On the one hand, where there is genuinely mental illness, the patient's expressed wishes about treatment may well not be rational. It is part of the very nature of what we call serious mental disorder that those who suffer from it lose their autonomy, their capacity to make rational decisions about at least some aspects of their lives. For the same reason, it may be unlikely that exploration of the patient's alleged reasons for their choice of treatment (or non-treatment) will result in those reasons becoming more intelligible, let alone coming to be seen as more rational. The only rational choice of treatment in such circumstances is the one which is most likely to lead to a restoration of the patient's autonomy. Yet the patient's present lack of autonomy does not mean that she is unworthy of respect for her humanity. Thus, respect for the patient as a human being must be distinguished from respect for autonomy, if that means acceptance of her current decisions about treatment. It consists rather in acting in what can be seen to be her best interests, even if this is against her will. Once again, this is not paternalistic if it is genuinely based on what she would see as in her best interests if she were genuinely autonomous, and the safeguards already mentioned (advance directives, etc.) can be applied in order to make this more likely. Yet there is also a further safeguard: no treatment can be ethically acceptable if it actually *prevents* her return to full autonomy, as for example certain kinds of brain surgery such as lobotomy might be seen as doing. (Though in very rare cases, even these treatments might be justifiable as a lesser evil, if they prevent some even greater harm to a patient.)

However there is a further complication in the psychiatric field: respect for the potential patient's humanity also requires sensitive exploration of the feelings behind the patient's initial choice of treatment. Such exploration may make it clear that the patient's decision is not as unintelligible as it first seemed: either because the patient's behaviour is not in fact disordered, but a reasonable response to a difficult situation, or because the patient's disorder does not affect her capacity to make decisions about the particular matter in hand. At the very least, psychiatrists owe it to their patients, as fellow human beings, to recognise that they may have feelings about particular aspects of the proposed treatment which need to be taken into account. The treatment in general may still be ethically required, but it can be applied in a more sensitive way. In all these ways, what is required in psychiatric ethics (and, I would say, in medical ethics generally) is not so much respect for patient autonomy as respect for the patient as a fellow human being, whose worth depends on all aspects of her humanity and not only on her (perhaps absent) power of rational decision-making.

References

BEAUCHAMP, T.L. & J.F. CHILDRESS, *Principles of Biomedical Ethics*, 5th edition, New York, Oxford University Press, 2001.

MATTHEWS, E., 'Autonomy and the Psychiatric Patient' in *Journal of Applied Philosophy* 17(2000), p. 1.

MILL, J.S., *On Liberty and Other Essays*, ed. J. GRAY, Oxford, Oxford University Press, 1998.

6. A BRIDGE OVER TROUBLED WATER
Paternalism as the Expression of Autonomy

Thomas Nys

It is difficult to reach common ground in the discussions on autonomy and paternalism. The concepts are frequently used and they appear in a wide variety of contexts. Even in the philosophical literature it seems that we have as many concepts of autonomy and paternalism as there are people working on the topic. Nevertheless, in spite of this complexity and confusion, there seems to be a remarkable underlying normative consensus which cuts across these differences. This consensus is quite straightforward: autonomy is something valuable[1], whereas paternalism is in need of justification. Autonomy is envisaged as a capacity, condition, or property which should be developed, protected and promoted while paternalism is tarnished with suspicion.[2] Joel Feinberg rightly notes that we normally *accuse* a person of paternalism[3], thereby indicating that it is

---

[1] "About the only feature held constant from one author to another is that autonomy is a feature of persons and that it is a desirable quality to have." G. DWORKIN, *The Theory and Practice of Autonomy*, Cambridge, Cambridge University Press, 1988, pp. 54-55.

[2] It is important to emphasise what I am *not* saying here. I am not saying that paternalism is *always* bad and that autonomy is *always* good. I am instead saying that paternalism is commonly held to be wrong *to the extent* that it violates something good, autonomy. Perhaps paternalism is also morally suspicious because it interferes with other valuable goods (like liberty, or perhaps more specific moral rules like rules against deceit or force), but at least autonomy is among the usual suspects. It should be clear that the definition of paternalism which I will discuss does not run afoul of the 'definitional stop': paternalism according to Dworkin is not necessarily illegitimate or morally wrong. Still, I want to discuss this descriptive, neutral account of paternalism in light of our moral convictions, i.e. in light of our general concern for autonomy, and show that while the first two of its conditions indicate the importance of the autonomy of the 'victim', the third points to the autonomy of the paternalist.

[3] J. FEINBERG, *Harm to Self: The Moral Limits of the Criminal Law*, New York, Oxford University Press, 1986, p. 4.

somehow insulting to be labelled with the paternalist mark: it is something one should be ashamed of.

If we try to explain what could account for the opposite valuations of autonomy and paternalism, we notice that the negative valuation of the second is the flip-side of the positive attitude toward the first: paternalism is 'bad' because it endangers the value of autonomy. Intuitively, this seems to make sense. Paternalist interventions prohibit a person to be self-reliant and self-determining, i.e. to exercise control over his own life and to live it the way he sees fit. Hence, autonomy and paternalism are commonly perceived as enemy notions; they relate to each other only as opposite sides of a coin.

In this paper I want to reconsider this dichotic perception. I do not want to contest the idea that paternalism goes against the value of autonomy, but I want to suggest that it is perhaps possible to bridge the gap between both concepts by arguing that paternalist actions and motives are often rooted in the autonomy of the paternalist. Such an approach, I maintain, has various advantages. Most importantly, it allows us to understand the ambiguous character of paternalism and it enables us to transcend the prevailing scenario in which autonomy systematically tends to triumph over paternalism.

1. Paternalism

Let us take a closer look at the concept of paternalism by focusing on a definition which, although neutral in itself, fits the underlying normative consensus by maintaining a tension with autonomy. This is the definition as it was developed by Gerald Dworkin in the *Stanford Encyclopedia of Philosophy*.[4] The definition, at least as I see it, stipulates three necessary conditions for paternalism; conditions which, if they are jointly fulfilled, are also sufficient. The definition goes as follows:

> X acts paternalistically towards Y by doing (omitting) Z if:
> Z (or its omission) interferes with the liberty or autonomy of Y
> X does so without the consent of Y, and
> X does so because Z will improve the welfare of Y (where this includes preventing his welfare from diminishing), or in some way promote the interests, values, or good of Y

---

[4] G. DWORKIN, 'Paternalism' in *The Stanford Encyclopedia of Philosophy* (2002) on http://plato.stanford.edu/archives/win 2002/entries/paternalism.

I will discuss the first two conditions and show how they relate to the normative consensus; I will then turn to the last condition and argue that although it is central to our understanding of paternalism, it is also the most troublesome feature.

The first condition, i.e. the action interferes with the liberty or autonomy of the victim, already suggests that there is a conflict with autonomy. This however, is not entirely correct because the condition contains a disjunction: paternalist actions violate a person's autonomy *or* his liberty. Put differently, there are certain paternalist interventions which infringe upon a person's liberty without violating his autonomy. But how should we understand this?

One way to make sense of this is to say that restrictions of (negative) liberty occur on the level of actions, whereas violations of autonomy take place on the level of desires or volitions. Infringements of liberty prevent a person from pursuing certain courses of action which he wants or might want to pursue, while infringements of autonomy try to modify, manipulate or change a person's desires. For example, if I lie to you and tell you that you don't have the required ability to join the local football team (although I am in fact extremely jealous of your exquisite technique), then I might prevent you from applying. My acts of deception can result in you wrongly believing that you wouldn't stand a chance. Now of course, I do not really (i.e. physically) prevent you from applying: you are as free as you were before. I only changed the way in which you perceived your opportunities. If you wanted to apply you could still go ahead, but I made sure that you do not want to do that anymore.[5]

Put differently, liberty is about the link between preferences and action: a person is free if he is able to do what he wants to do, that is, if he is able to translate his desires into actions (when he is allowed to 'go ahead'). A violation of liberty is to prevent a person from doing what he wants to do. Autonomy, on Dworkin's account, is the capacity for forming second-order desires by means of critical reflection. A violation of autonomy would therefore mean, I believe, that one

---

[5] This is an attempt to identify a situation in which a person's autonomy is violated *without* his freedom being interfered with. However, it is not clear what Dworkin's position on this matter would be. It is clear that the condition of 'procedural independence' is meant to prevent practices such as hypnosis or neurological manipulation from determining the will of an autonomous person, but it leaves the question of whether deceit really by-passes a person's capacity for critical reflection. I will come back to the difficulty of interfering with a person's autonomy in section 3.

distorts, disrupts or otherwise tampers with the process of critical reflection, for instance, through by-passing the mechanism by means of hypnosis or brainwashing (i.e. by violating what Dworkin calls the condition of 'procedural independence'). Such cases of paternalism seem to be very rare. Yet, perhaps the violation need not be so strong. Deception, for example, might be a case in point. We can imagine that a man who hides his sleeping pills because he is afraid that his wife will commit suicide does not prevent her from doing what she wants to do, for there are many ways to take one's own life. Instead, what he tries to avoid is that his wife's desire for suicide will be triggered by being confronted with these pills. Hence, he tries to avoid her desire for suicide from coming to the surface. Although he does not really manipulate or coerce her, the act of deception still operates on the level of desires, or more precisely, on the level of desire-formation.

Now, can there be cases of paternalism in which someone interferes with another person's liberty (i.e. he prevents her from doing what she wants) without, on the one hand, tampering with the agent's capacity for critical reflection and, on the other hand, without preventing her from carrying out her reflectively endorsed desires (because the most common way of interfering with a person's autonomy is by means of an infringement of liberty)? Perhaps. Suppose that someone has decided to stop smoking but that when cramming for his exams, he is so caught up in the moment that he automatically puts a cigarette in his mouth. Now suppose that another person, his roommate, sees this and prevents him from lighting the cigarette. Is this a case of paternalism? His liberty is in fact infringed, and he has not consented, but the desires which are externally frustrated by his roommate are not autonomous desires, but alienating ones; desires which he has repudiated on a higher level after critical reflection. Such paternalism, although it exists, is also less troublesome. So, although the definition puts them on a par (liberty and autonomy), it seems that the less the interference goes against a person's autonomy, the less it can be called paternalist.

The same goes for the second condition. Why is consent so important? Why is it even mentioned in the definition? Well, because we believe that it reveals something about a person's autonomy. We think of consent as a reliable indicator of a person's true wishes and preferences. Perhaps what a person says and tells us about these desires is not the only indicator[6] but it certainly counts as a prominent source of information. Consequently, we do not value consent (or we value it less) if it is not 'backed up' by autonomy, for example, if it is only the expression of superficial or whimsical desires. Again, the consent condition becomes more important the more it reveals something about a person's 'real self'.

Not only do the first two conditions tell us what an act should be like in order to be called 'paternalist', it also shows how accusations of paternalism can be avoided. As such, it reveals two important *evasive strategies*. The first strategy is to argue for the non-autonomy of the victim because one cannot interfere with what a person does not have. Competence, for example, is generally perceived as a necessary condition for autonomy, so if a person lacks competence, he also lacks autonomy. But what is competence? In psychiatry and mental health care, competence tests are commonly used, but these tests are far from uniform and universal. They range from very mild and lenient tests — e.g., is the person capable of making a choice? — to very severe tests — does the patient understand all the relevant information and can he defend his choice by means of rational argument? Some authors have argued that these instruments are themselves used paternalistically, or better, that they are used to cover up paternalist concerns.[7] Doctors apply severe competence tests if they disagree with their patient's decisions and they use weak tests in cases where their patient agrees with them. If this is true, then these assessments of competence are merely used as instruments of justification.

The second condition reveals another evasive strategy: the highly popular *search for consent*. In order to avoid accusations of paternalism, the paternalist has to show that his victim has somehow consented to the interference. However, there are many different kinds of consent and because the definition leaves it unspecified which kind is relevant, it allows leeway for evasion. For example, we can distinguish between actual, prior, subsequent, proxy, and hypothetical consent. Although actual consent is fairly unproblematic, prior

---

[6] Robert Young mentions remorse as another indicator for revealing a person's true wishes. We feel remorse when we have betrayed our true self. See R. YOUNG, 'Compatibilism and Conditioning' in *Noûs* 13(1979), pp. 36-46.

[7] L. ROTH et al., 'Tests of Competency to Consent to Treatment' in *American Journal of Psychiatry* 134(1977), pp. 279-284.

consent already has to deal with the difficulty that a person might have changed his mind. Subsequent consent is perhaps even more dubious because, as Kasachkoff has put it, "gratitude does not make it okay".[8] The paternalist intervention might have an effect on a person's subsequent consent (e.g., brainwashing). Also, the legitimacy of proxy consent is endangered by the fact that the proxies might not (or cannot) totally detach from their own perspective and therefore might act paternalistically themselves. And last but not least, hypothetical consent might start from a hypothesis which has little bearing upon the actual person. For example, it could start from the assumption of a perfectly rational decision maker. Therefore, correspondingly to the use of competence tests, the search for consent is primarily a means of justification.

Now let us turn to the third condition. This criterion deserves special attention because it seems to reveal a positive aspect of paternalism. Whereas the first two conditions are often invoked to express what is wrong with paternalism, the third seems to attenuate the dubious character of such interventions since the purpose of paternalism is to ameliorate the welfare of the individual. This aspect however, is often neglected or insufficiently understood. According to the definition, for example, many of the actions which we call paternalistic in everyday practice are, in fact, not paternalist at all. When a company insists that its employees should wear safety helmets then the motive for this precautionary matter is probably purely selfish. The company needs a healthy staff in order to be productive and accidents would therefore severely cut into its profits. Also, in many cases interventions are intended to prevent *harm to others* instead of harm to self. When we insist that heroin addicts should receive mandatory treatment, we may wonder whether we do so for the sake of these addicts or simply because we think that it is better or safer for *us* or for *others* to keep them off the streets. These considerations make it clear that the class of paternalist actions is presumably smaller than we believe. In fact, the class might very well be empty if the third condition is *never* fulfilled.

The condition states that the paternalist act should improve the welfare of its victim, but it leaves unspecified from what perspective this well-being should be perceived. Initially, it seems to make sense if we

---

[8] T. KASACHKOFF, 'Paternalism: Does Gratitude Make It Okay?' in *Social Theory and Practice* 20(1994), pp. 1-23.

interpret 'well-being' in objective terms: e.g., we know that it is better to be without a swollen appendix and therefore a doctor might feel justified in 'repairing' this deficiency without the patient's explicit consent. However, such an objective account comes at a price and what initially seemed to be a 'positive aspect' quickly becomes suspicious.

John Stuart Mill mentions the famous example of a person who is about to cross an unsafe bridge.[9] According to Mill, we are allowed (and even obliged!) to stop this person because it is reasonable to believe that he is simply unaware of the danger: we assume that his intention is to cross the bridge safely and not that he wants to plummet into the water. Now, suppose that we make the reasonable assumption that it is better for a human being to be alive rather than dead,[10] then it seems that we should stop this man *regardless* of his preferences. Whether he is competent or not, whether he has consented or not, that doesn't matter: he should be stopped to preserve his objective well-being. This is a clear case of (hard) paternalism, and it is often believed to be objectionable because it ignores an important aspect of well-being.[11] The underlying idea is that a person's welfare is at least partially dependent upon first-person considerations. People have different commitments and these commitments determine the boundaries of their welfare. Perceived as such, it is quite understandable that people are willing to sacrifice their objective well-being in order to protect the things they care about. A loving parent, for example, might choose to sacrifice her own life in order to prevent her children from suffering serious misfortune. But these personal commitments, as the term suggests, are far from universal, let alone objective.

However, if we incorporate the first-person perspective as a necessary ingredient, that is to say, if we indeed believe that the individual is the final judge concerning his own well-being, then the notion of (hard) paternalism stops making any sense.[12] How can the

[9]   J.S. MILL, *On Liberty*, ed. M. WARNOCK, Malden, MA, Blackwell Publishing, 2003, p. 165.

[10] See the contribution of Eric Matthews in this volume (p. 135).

[11] In fact, a lot of paternalism is justified by referring to an objective account of well-being i.e. one that is independent of an agent's desires and preferences.

[12] What if the paternalist uses a desire-satisfaction theory of well-being (I owe this suggestion to Ishtiyaque Haji)? Insofar as desires and their satisfaction are dependent upon the first-person perspective, it is difficult to grasp how the third condition could ever be jointly fulfilled with the first two conditions of Dworkin's definition. For example it seems unlikely, yet perhaps not totally inconceivable, that someone would take care of an individual's desires (by making sure that they are satisfied) without

paternalist be genuinely concerned about the well-being of his 'victims' if he disregards their own wishes, if he disregards the closest approximation of their well-being, i.e. their consent? If he really cared about their welfare then he would allow them to steer their own course. For sure, people are sometimes mistaken about their true preferences, but after due inquiry, the ultimate responsibility should lay with the individual. To come back to the example of Mill: if the person who is about to cross an unsafe bridge tells us that his intention is to commit suicide, then, on this account, we would have to let him go.[13] What could possibly motivate our interference? Surely, it cannot be the excuse of caring about *his* well-being. Thus, on this interpretation, the third condition for paternalism strikes us as insincere. The 'paternalist' must have a hidden agenda: there must be some concealed self-interest or, considered from a more favourable perspective, a wish to prevent harm to others. Though, whatever his intention might be, it is not a genuine concern to prevent so-called 'harm to self'. Therefore, in order to make sense of paternalism, we should seek to combine the idea that a paternalist applies a conception of the good which is independent from that of its victim (hence, the possibility of conflict) and the requirement that the paternalist motive indeed expresses a genuine concern for the individual's well-being.

2. Love

In this section I want to present an interpretation of the third condition which is able to combine these ideas. In order to understand how this condition operates, let us focus on an exemplar: the way parents treat their children. It is important to note that our common, everyday use of the term 'paternalism' has shifted in the sense that it is now used to express an analogy: someone acts paternalistically

---

obtaining their consent for this interference. The point is that whenever the paternalist makes his conception of well-being dependent upon the individual, the danger of paternalism diminishes. The clash with autonomy becomes less acute.

[13] It should be noted however, that this conclusion does not immediately follow from Mill's discussion of soft paternalism. In *On Liberty* he starts from the assumption that the individual does *not* want to die, and he does not mention the scenario of suicide. He only says that we should let this person cross the bridge if he thinks it is safe (and the end-result might indeed be that the bridge collapses).

if he treats a competent, adult human being *as if* she were a child. Such behaviour is demeaning and patronising. Again, this common interpretation leaves little room for uncontested paternalism: an act is either paternalist and demeaning, or it is not paternalist at all. As a result of this interpretation, we only seldom accuse parents of behaving paternalistically towards their children. However, what tends to get snowed under by this interpretation is that the paternalist is committed to a very demanding position. The things a parent does for his children, or at least the things that he *believes* he should do, go well beyond the requirements he has towards other people (e.g., complete strangers).[14] Their well-being means more to him in the sense that it has a bearing on his own personal welfare. He is somehow 'emotionally invested' in his children.

Likewise, if there is indeed such a thing as 'moral distance'[15], then it seems as if the paternalist includes its 'victims' in a close, or at least closer, perimeter. He really takes the well-being of these persons to heart in the sense that he is anything but indifferent. Now, if the paternalist attitude is indeed quite the opposite of indifference, an attitude which we hold in contempt, then it seems that at least *that* aspect of paternalism is praiseworthy and that it should be encouraged.

Nevertheless, it is important to note that in taking care of his children, a loving parent does not detach from his own perspective, i.e. he strives to improve *their* well-being in a way which *he* deems appropriate. A father might prevent his child from stuffing himself with sweets, and this 'forceful intervention' is indeed paternalistic because the child has no desire whatsoever to refrain from eating sweets. He just wants all the sweets he can get his little hands on. Hence, parents do not act upon the presupposition that their children

---

[14] This does not imply that all paternalist acts are supererogatory, i.e. that they do more than is morally required (although this is often the case with parents). Some parents, although they are genuinely concerned about the well-being of their children, are in fact very poor caretakers. Still, even bad parents are not indifferent to the welfare of their offspring; they just have a warped view of what that well-being consists in. Now, insofar as morality implies the overcoming of indifference, the condition of 'caring about' is a prelude to morality. Hence, it should be clear that paternalism is not necessarily good, but at least it expresses a pre-moral commitment: one is not insensitive to the well-being of another person; one truly cares.

[15] J. GLOVER, *Causing Death and Saving Lives*, New York, Penguin Books, 1979; R. ABELSON, 'Moral Distance: What Do We Owe To Unknown Strangers?' in *The Philosophical Forum* 16(2005), pp. 31-39.

have a hidden and 'true' desire for healthy nutrition. Perhaps they want to instil such a desire, but the scheme of education is still very different from the act of paternalism, viz. the blunt prohibition of (too many) sweets. Thus the conception of well-being which parents use in taking care of their offspring is *their* conception, not that of their children. Of course, they might be sensitive to their child's wishes and preferences, but ultimately, parents put their foot down whenever the pursuit of these preferences gets out of hand.

A proper account of paternalism requires that we move beyond the 'soft' and careful idea of translation and transparency.[16] For example, it requires that we concentrate on the hard paternalism which underlies the evasive strategies. Such paternalism, I claim, is based upon the exemplar of parental concern and, as such, it is an ambiguous concept: an intricate combination of (and tension between) *maternal love* and *paternal resoluteness*.[17]

However, the fact that paternalism can be explained as an act of love is generally neglected. We might be willing to give parents the benefit of the doubt, but it surely seems wildly exaggerated to invoke the concept of love when we discuss the relationship between doctors and patients. Doctors do not love their patients except perhaps in fairytales and soap operas.[18] Moreover, we believe that doctors do

---

[16] The dominance of the transparency model, i.e. the idea that we should honour *only* the patient's wishes and that we should therefore try to reveal *his* true preferences, is also apparent in the proposed standards for dealing with incompetent patients. Consider, for example, the *substituted judgment principle* "which directs the surrogate to use available knowledge of the patient and his or her values and wishes to attempt to decide as the patient would have decided in the circumstances that now obtain if the patient were competent." The ideal of transparency is also paramount in the *pure autonomy standard* which "applies exclusively to formerly autonomous, now incompetent patients who expressed a relevant autonomous preference. This standard specifies the general commitments of the principle of respect for autonomy. One must respect the past, self-regarding, autonomous decisions reached by now-incompetent but previously competent persons". Both accounts involve an attempt to approximate the preferences of the now-incompetent patient. Only the *best interests standard* allows for true paternalism. See T.L. BEAUCHAMP & J.F. CHILDRESS, *Principles of Biomedical Ethics*, 5th edition, New York, Oxford University Press, 2001, p. 99.

[17] Perhaps the gender-related terms (maternal, paternal) are used in an outdated and even sexist way, thereby confirming the stereotypical roles of men and women. I do not endorse such stereotypes and I certainly do not want to encourage them. Still, I am always at a loss when figuring out what kind of phrasing would be 'politically correct'.

[18] The common objection is that doctors should *take care of* their patients instead of *caring about* them. It is clear that a doctor can provide adequate care for his patients for a host of different reasons (duty, money, prestige, fun...). Put differently, 'caring

not *need* to love their patients.[19] After all, they get paid rather well for their services. However, if a serious account of paternalism entails an aspect of love, if genuine paternalism is based upon the model of parental love, then the result in the context of health care seems to be straightforward: there is no love and therefore no paternalism. Or else: if there is indeed paternalism, then it is certainly not rooted in love.

Love however, can be quite modest. It does not necessarily imply sweaty hands, eternal commitments, and acts of folly or total self-effacement. I can love my dog, chocolate fudge, or basketball games and neither of these loves need to go particularly deep. Throughout the past thirty-five years, Harry Frankfurt has developed an interesting account of the phenomenon of love. In fact, Frankfurt's concept of love is an elaboration, a sub-category so to speak, of his earlier analysis of 'caring about something'.[20] With regard to his earlier concept, Frankfurt made clear that persons are often moved to action out of a concern for 'the things they care about'. Hence, as a

for' does not presuppose 'caring about'. A doctor, for example, can care for his patients like a mechanic takes care of a customer's car. He improves the condition of this car simply because it is his job, i.e. because that is what he gets paid for. If he is a 'bad' mechanic, customers will not return. This however, does not imply that he cares about these cars or their owners. At the end of the day, he only cares about his pay cheque. Note that the mechanic's (doctor's) autonomous actions are still rooted in his 'caring about something', only now he cares about the money instead of the car. What the mechanic does to the car is only a means to achieve his ultimate goal; his well-being is not directly linked to that of the car (he wouldn't be a mechanic if he won the lottery). If this is true for the relationship between patients and caretakers, i.e. they care for them because they care about something different, then we could wonder what all the fuss is about. Why would these caretakers persist if their well-being is not directly affected by the condition of their patients? Like the mechanic, they could take care of the patient in whatever way the patient (customer) sees fit. However, if the reasons for paternalism are other than a disinterested concern in the victim's well-being then we seem to lose the meaning of the concept. It is precisely my point that we have difficulties in understanding the concept of paternalism. For some important limits of my analysis, see section 3 below.

[19] I will come to the objection that doctors *should* not love their patients in section 3.

[20] For the similarities between both concepts, see H. Frankfurt, *Necessity, Volition, and Love*, Cambridge, Cambridge University Press, 1999, p. 129; H. Frankfurt, *The Reasons of Love*, Princeton, NJ, Princeton University Press, 2004, p. 31. The distinctive feature of love is that it is a *disinterested concern* for the things one cares about. One could care about something as a means to an end, while the well-being of the things one loves is always a goal in itself. Another difference is that love is essentially *personal*, i.e. the object of love is "ineluctably particular". See H. Frankfurt, *The Reasons of Love*, pp. 42-44.

source of motivation 'caring about something' is at least as important as the commands of moral duty.[21]

Frankfurt mentions several features of love and I will discuss only a few of them. First, the objects of our love are not self-chosen. We are somehow captivated by the things we love[22]; they pick us and we respond. Secondly, there is no conceptual limit as to the possible content of the things we care about.

> [T]he range of potential objects of care is itself extremely wide and diverse. One may care about oneself, other people (or simply the plight of other people), animals (or simply the plight of animals), the environment, how one is treated, peace on earth, works of art (and beautiful things in general), God, fictional characters, morality, one's nation, one's ideals, and even other of one's cares. And this is just the tip of the iceberg.[23]

Such content-neutrality means that even silly things or things which we deem unworthy of love can nevertheless be objects of care.

Third, *in* loving or *through* loving, a person connects his well-being to the well-being of the things he loves. Thereby he makes himself vulnerable to the gains and losses, the ups and downs, of his beloveds. For example, a true and committed football fan will feel miserable if his team loses. Yet, and this is fundamental, love entails a disinterested concern for the beloved, that is to say, the welfare of the object of love takes priority over the welfare of the lover: "For the lover, the condition of his beloved is important in itself, apart from any bearing that it may have on other matters".[24] Love is never merely instrumental.

3. Autonomy

What is interesting is that the concept of 'caring about' is fundamental in Frankfurt's analysis of autonomy. It truly is fundamental in the

---

[21] For an extremely lucid discussion of the differences between Kant's account of autonomy and Frankfurt's, see H. FRANKFURT, *Necessity, Volition, and Love*, Cambridge, Cambridge University Press, 1999, pp. 129-141.

[22] H. FRANKFURT, *Necessity, Volition, and Love*, p. 135.

[23] D. SHOEMAKER, 'Caring, Identification, and Agency' in *Ethics* 114(2003), p. 94.

[24] H. FRANKFURT, *The Reasons of Love*, p. 42.

sense that it solves the problems of internality and authority.[25] Frankfurt is well-known for his distinction between first- and second-order desires: a person enjoys autonomy if his will, i.e. the first-order desires which actually move him to action, corresponds to his higher-order volitions. For example, a smoker only smokes out of his own free will if he is satisfied with his desire (read: urge) for a cigarette; that is, if he wants to be moved by this desire. But, if first-order desires are rendered autonomous by being backed up by corresponding higher-order desires, then what establishes the autonomy of these higher desires? How can we avoid the danger of infinite regress? And secondly, what is the status of these volitions? The problem is that they *remain* desires, a feature which makes them too weak or volatile to grant any authority (as opposed to desires backed up by *reasons*, for example). In short, it seems to be a theory without solid foundations.

To solve these problems, Frankfurt points to the reality of what he calls the 'necessities of the will'. Sometimes a person is confronted with the boundaries of his will. These are moments in which he realises that he cannot will otherwise. Now if these boundaries are indeed given and not self-created, that is, not under the agent's direct control, then it is possible to put an end to the threatening infinite regress of ever higher orders of desires. The concept of necessities of the will also solves the problem of authority because these necessities are *constitutive* of a person's identity. But how should we understand this?

Frankfurt gives the example of Martin Luther who famously said: "Here I stand, I cannot do otherwise". In making this statement, Luther declared that he experienced a certain necessity of his will. Of course, he did not really have to take a stand: nobody forced him to defend the protestant creed (much to the contrary!). Neither was he swept away by an overwhelming alienating desire. Luther did what he did because he wanted to do so. The fact that he couldn't bring himself to do anything different was not due to a lack of will-power, but to the composure of his will itself. He deeply *identified* with whatever it was that he felt he had to do. This indicates that such necessities determine the 'contours of agency'; they are constitutive of a person's volitional identity, of his character, of who he is and who he

---

[25] S. CUYPERS, 'Autonomy beyond Voluntarism: In Defense of Hierarchy' in *Canadian Journal of Philosophy* 30(2000), pp. 225-256.

wants to be. They enjoy authority because they have a hold on the individual, i.e. they transcend his immediate control, while, on a deeper level, they precisely determine the preconditions for control. Hence, a person lacks control if he cannot do justice to his volitional necessities.

But where do these necessities come from? According to Frankfurt they are the result of 'caring about' or loving something. Luther only took his stand because he deeply cared about his ideals. In fact, you cannot claim to love something or somebody if you do not experience some volitional necessity with regard to them. As I said before, love entails that the lover has connected his fate to that of his beloved. This implies that he is summoned to action if the well-being of the things he loves is seriously endangered: he is then faced with what Frankfurt calls the *unthinkable*. There are just some things that a person cannot allow to happen to his loved ones. He then feels that he must act — or that he should refrain from action — in order to protect or promote their well-being. If there is no such point at which the lover is spurred to action, then there is no true love.

In this regard, Frankfurt mentions a woman who realises that she is unable to give her child up for adoption.[26] Like in Luther's case, there is no external force because nobody prevents this woman from doing anything: in terms of negative liberty, she is perfectly free. However, this mother feels that she would fail herself if she signs the adoption forms. She does not want to be that kind of person; she does not want to be the abandoning mother. Now what would happen if we forced this woman to sign these forms after all? In a strict sense we cannot violate her autonomy because she might still be moved — unsuccessfully though — by her authentic desire to refrain from signing. Nevertheless, we could say that we do not *respect* her autonomy. Desires are always aimed at action and therefore, respect for autonomy would mean very little if we did not allow for this translation into action. What is the point of discriminating between true and false preferences if the boundaries of action are already externally fixed? To allow for personal autonomy as a feature of the human will (i.e. the correspondence of lower-order desires and higher-order volitions) is insufficient. For we could imagine situations in which individuals are

---

[26] G. WATSON, 'Volitional Necessities' in S. BUSS & L. OVERTON (eds.), *Contours of Agency: Essays on Themes from Harry Frankfurt*, Cambridge, MIT Press, 2002, pp. 129-160.

perfectly free to want whatever they want to want, but in which they should do whatever *we* want them to *do*. This is the liberty of the frustrated slave who is free to have all the wishes and dreams he can imagine while, at the same time, he sees himself shackled in chains and locks.[27] This is autonomy captured in tears; freedom expressed in the dull sound of fists banging on prison walls. One sees oneself motivated by the appropriate desires, but unable to bring these desires into action. Such freedom is hypocritical and cheap.

What matters for our present purpose is that Frankfurt, in the mother-adoption example, mentions parental love in the context of autonomy. Not only are volitional necessities perfectly compatible with autonomy, they are also *essential*. David Shoemaker has convincingly shown that all autonomous action is ultimately rooted in volitional necessity.[28] This implies that all of our autonomous desires can be traced back to the things we care about.[29] Thus, if we accept that we cannot make sense of paternalism without the concept of love (because of the intertwinement of the lover's well-being with that of his beloved), and if we accept that love is not only compatible with, but also constitutive of a person's autonomy, then the paternalist motive is ultimately rooted in the autonomy of the paternalist. To be able to be moved by caring desires is to be autonomous. To be able to translate this 'caring about' into action, i.e. into 'taking care of the things one cares about', is to be respected in one's autonomy.

Perhaps it is helpful to take a look at the ground we have covered so far. We have argued that genuine paternalism hinges upon a condition which seems unintelligible. We no longer understand what it means to care about another person's well-being while disregarding their own preferences. Therefore, in order to make the third condition intelligible, we have referred to an important exemplar: the parent-child relationship. Conceived as such, 'paternalism' is essentially an ambiguous concept: it is a combination of paternal resoluteness (the

---

[27] This is different from the Stoic slave who is satisfied with his lot. Although we would also hesitate to call this genuine freedom, we could perhaps agree that the fate of the frustrated slave is even worse.

[28] D. SHOEMAKER, 'Caring, Identification, and Agency', pp. 88-118.

[29] Perhaps some people would feel that this is exaggerated because many of our actions do not refer to the things we care about. Shoemaker however, would agree. At many times we are perfectly indifferent about our will; we happily follow the economy of our desires (we then behave non-autonomously, or 'wantonlike' in Frankfurt's vocabulary).

independence of the conception of the good which is imposed) and maternal love (an unconditional concern for the well-being of the child). Yet, if love is indeed necessary to account for paternalism then it does not seem to exist in the medical context: doctors do not really love their patients. We then proposed a modest account of love based on Harry Frankfurt's explorations of what it means to care about something. We have shown how love relates to the necessities of the will, and in what sense love is essential to autonomy. Paradoxically, self-determination only makes sense against a background of caring about something other than the self. The autonomous person is able to live his life according to the 'commands of love': he is respected in his autonomy if he is able to go wherever his love may lead him. Our conclusion is that at least some instances of paternalism are rooted in autonomy (e.g., the autonomy of parents in caring about their children). In fact, and this is a much stronger claim, paternalism only makes sense if we refer to the autonomy of the paternalist[30], that is, if we understand the connection between his welfare and that of whom he cares about.

Despite the fact that in many cases paternalism finds its origin in the autonomy of the paternalist, we should note that this conclusion remains rather moderate. Our analysis only shows that paternalists — say doctors — *could* claim respect for their autonomy *if* they refer to the necessities of their will which, in turn, are the result of their truly caring about the welfare of their patients. First of all, this requires that paternalists should be willing to defend that they care about their patients, that is, that they provide care for these individuals *because* they care about them. Perhaps not many doctors are willing to defend that they are somehow emotionally invested in the condition of their patients. It seems that doctors should always keep their professional distance and that they shouldn't get involved too much. Nevertheless, this does not imply that they shouldn't get involved at all.[31] In my opinion, if doctors could sincerely point out that they love their patients in a non-tacky way, i.e. that they are engaged in the things they truly care about, sometimes even to the extent that their necessities of the will come into play, *then* they could also claim respect for their autonomy.

---

[30] Actually, Frankfurt does not discuss the autonomy of persons, only the autonomy of desires. What we mean when we use the expression 'the autonomy of the paternalist' is that he is able to be motivated by the things he cares about.

[31] See the contribution of George Agich in this volume (p. 83).

4. Restoring the Balance

Where does this analysis lead us? Well, essentially it does not solve any problems at all. Much to the contrary: it reveals a central quandary. Yet I believe that it is better to have real problems than easy solutions in this respect. Let me explain this.

At the outset of this paper I mentioned a remarkable consensus: the "good-bad" dichotomy with regard to autonomy and paternalism. This implies that whenever the autonomy of patients is balanced against the alleged paternalist intentions of doctors or care-takers, i.e. intentions which go against the preferences of the patient, autonomy is believed to win by default. Hence, there is no real conflict: either the care-taker has to take a step back and respect the autonomy of the patient, or he tries to cover up his motivations by means of various evasive strategies. Whichever direction one takes, real (hard) paternalism is considered anathema.

In order to restore the balance, we have to give the paternalist his voice back. This chapter was intended to explore how we could achieve such a goal by showing that a caring paternalist can rightfully claim respect for his autonomy as well. Perhaps many people would object that the patient has much more to lose (e.g., his life and limbs) than the paternalist (a mere insult to his feelings of superiority), but I believe that such an objection is foolhardy. The content of the desire is irrelevant to the question of autonomy. Moreover, Frankfurt's conception of autonomy erases any clear distinction between one's proper well-being and that of the things one cares about. Autonomy is always directed outwards. In a liberal society we are eager to employ rather weak and formal conditions for autonomy (i.e. it is not *what* a person wants, but the *way in which* he holds these desires). This fits our predicament of pluralism. For Frankfurt this even implies that the question of morality should be treated independently from the descriptive question of autonomy. However, Frankfurt never maintained that such a normative discussion, i.e. what are the things that we *should* care about, should never take place. Some instances of autonomy should clearly be rejected as immoral (e.g., Hitler's autonomy). Now, in my opinion, one can either opt for a thick concept of autonomy which incorporates a certain 'moral minimum'[32], or else one could employ a thin descriptive

---

[32] See, for instance, O. ONEILL, *Autonomy and Trust in Bioethics*, Cambridge, Cambridge University Press, 2002.

concept of personal autonomy which is insufficient to warrant moral respect (because a person might care about the wrong things). These days however, it seems that we have opted for the idea that weak autonomy is sufficient for a person to demand moral respect. This avoids a clash between different instances of autonomy (e.g., multiculturalism), but it also avoids a substantial discussion on the good life.

The attempt to bridge the gap between autonomy and paternalism is a means to putting an end to the endless postponing of this substantial discussion. We should acknowledge that the real issue at hand is a confrontation between different conceptions of the good. For example, imagine a Jehovah's Witness who refuses an urgent blood transfusion. This person requests to die with dignity and he refers to deep-seated religious convictions to argue that his desires should be respected. On my account, a doctor might feel that he is unable to allow this unnecessary death. He experiences a necessity of his will; i.e. he cannot allow for this steep downfall in health and remain a passive bystander. This is not who he is and it is definitely not who he wants to be: he is a doctor, a caretaker and a life-saver. Consequently, he would fail himself if he lets this man die. This is no selfish concern because, not only would he fail himself, he would also fail his patient. His primary worry is the Jehovah's Witness. The doctor finds it difficult to acknowledge the value of these religious ideals. All he sees is a needless waste of life.

Now where does this leave us? Should the doctor insist, ignore the patient's wishes and condemn him to a life that he does not want to live? Or should he take a step back and keep his 'private concerns' to himself? Although I believe that the second strategy is dominant, I do not want to advocate the first. Instead I intend to encourage dialogue, but in order for this to be possible we have to acknowledge that there is conflict, real conflict that has to be addressed sooner or later, and preferably sooner than later. We need to find some common ground with regard to the good life. Of course, this normative (political, philosophical…) discussion should not take place at the bedside of a dying person. That would be far too late. However, I fully admit that I have no idea what shape this discussion should take and what the results will be. I can only say that a unilateral focus on the autonomy of the patient avoids any such discussion. Of course, paternalists might very well care about the wrong things, but we cannot know this in advance; it cannot be the default position that paternalists are always wrong. Both parties have to meet on equal grounds.

References

ABELSON, R., 'Moral Distance: What Do We Owe to Unknown Strangers?' in *The Philosophical Forum* 16(2005), pp. 31-39.

BEAUCHAMP, T.L. & J.F. CHILDRESS, *Principles of Biomedical Ethics*, 5th edition, New York, Oxford University Press, 2001.

CUYPERS, S., 'Autonomy beyond Voluntarism: In Defence of Hierarchy' in *Canadian Journal of Philosophy* 30(2000), pp. 225-256.

DWORKIN, G., *The Theory and Practice of Autonomy*, Cambridge, Cambridge University Press, 1988.

DWORKIN, G., 'The Concept of Autonomy' in J. CHRISTMAN (ed.), *The Inner Citadel: Essays on Individual Autonomy*, New York, Oxford University Press, 1989, pp. 54-62.

DWORKIN, G., 'Paternalism' in *The Stanford Encyclopedia of Philosophy* (2002) Retrieved Winter 2002, from http://plato.stanford.edu/archives/win2002/entries/paternalism

FEINBERG, J., *Harm to Self: The Moral Limits of the Criminal Law*, New York, Oxford University Press, 1986.

FRANKFURT, H., *Necessity, Volition, and Love*, Cambridge, Cambridge University Press, 1999.

FRANKFURT, H., *The Reasons of Love*, Princeton, NJ, Princeton University Press, 2004.

GLOVER, J., *Causing Death and Saving Lives*, New York, Penguin Books, 1979.

KASACHKOFF, T., 'Paternalism: Does Gratitude Make It Okay?' in *Social Theory and Practice* 20(1994), pp. 1-23.

MILL, J.S., *On Liberty*, ed. M. WARNOCK, Malden, Blackwell Publishing, 2003.

O'NEILL, O., *Autonomy and Trust in Bioethics*, Cambridge, Cambridge University Press, 2002.

ROTH, L.H., A. MEISEL & C.W. LIDZ, 'Tests of Competency to Consent to Treatment' in *American Journal of Psychiatry* 134(1977), pp. 279-284.

SHOEMAKER, D., 'Caring, Identification, and Agency' in *Ethics* 114(2003), pp. 88-118.

WATSON, G., 'Volitional Necessities' in S. BUSS & L. OVERTON (eds.), *Contours of Agency: Essays on Themes from Harry Frankfurt*, Cambridge, MIT Press, 2002, pp. 129-159.

7. AUTHORITY AND INFLUENCE IN THE PSYCHOTHERAPEUTIC RELATIONSHIP[1]

Heike Schmidt-Felzmann

Although psychotherapy is part of the health care system, it differs in important respects from other forms of health care. This has implications for understanding the challenges that therapists face with regard to the issue of paternalism. Paternalism in psychotherapy has an appearance that differs from the prototypical forms of paternalism discussed with regard to medical practice. These differences may have contributed to the perception of paternalism as an overall less serious ethical problem for psychotherapeutic practice. However, the apparent dissimilarities disguise problematic forms of interaction that should be understood as paternalistic. Psychotherapists themselves have addressed the problem of imposing their values on the patient since the early times of psychoanalysis and have developed strategies to counter illegitimate influence on the patient. However, as I will argue, those strategies are not only insufficient to solve the problem of paternalism, but the central place that they take within most therapeutic systems may lead to a kind of moral complacency and an underestimation of the extent to which hidden forms of illegitimate influence do in fact occur in the practice of therapy.

1. Anti-Paternalism in Psychotherapy

Discussions on paternalism in medical ethics so far have had little influence in the field of psychotherapy. This might be explained by

[1] I am grateful for the many comments and discussions on different aspects of this paper during the Leuven conference on Autonomy and Paternalism in May 2005, in particular the debate that was stimulated by the contributions of Gerald Dworkin and Eva Kittay.

the fact that prototypical characteristics of paternalism that are high-lighted in the medical ethics literature have little in common with the treatment situations that psychotherapists face. Cases that are fre-quently used in medical ethics to introduce the problem of paternal-ism refer, for example, to withholding information on the diagnosis of a fatal illness and treatment without the patient's knowledge or against the patient's expressed wishes. The most prominent ethical worries in relation to such decisions concern the patient's lack of knowledge of significant treatment information or the use of force or other modes of coercion. When described in these terms, these prob-lems do not seem likely to arise in the context of psychotherapy, at least with regard to voluntary outpatient therapy with adults, the most paradigmatic form of delivery of psychotherapy. Psychiatric diagnosis itself cannot proceed without communicating explicitly about the relevant problems, and unlike many medical interventions, psychotherapy cannot be administered to patients in a way that bypasses their awareness, understanding and consent. Just how con-siderable the differences between prototypical cases of paternalistic practice in medicine and psychotherapeutic practice are, is also reflected in the role given to the most popular antidote to paternalis-tic practice, namely informed consent procedures. While informed consent is one of the most prominent topics in medical ethics, and while training and medical practice nowadays is characterised by an extensive use of a variety of informed consent procedures, such pro-cedures have been developed only very recently in psychotherapy, and over and above fulfilling legal requirements, interest in the development of meaningful informed consent procedures is still rather limited in the psychotherapeutic community.

However, acknowledging these differences between medicine and psychotherapy is not tantamount to denying the importance of the problem of paternalism in psychotherapy. It neither means that con-ceptualisations of paternalism in medical ethics are entirely inapplic-able to psychotherapy, nor does it mean that psychotherapy has so far been oblivious to the ethical problem of paternalism. On the con-trary, whereas in medical ethics paternalism became only generally recognised as a problem in the 1970s, in psychotherapy, the impor-tance of problems related to paternalism has been acknowledged since the beginnings of modern psychotherapy at the end of the 19th century and has motivated the development of central therapeutic techniques and interventions. However, this attention to problems of paternalism has always been approached in fairly specific terms; the patient's interest in the process of therapy has not been taken too seriously, nor has much attention been paid to the concepts of coercion or deception in the specific conceptualisations of paternalism in psychotherapy. Instead, the main focus of attention has been the notion of "not interfering with patients' values".

The shortcomings of this traditional approach to the problem of paternalism in psychotherapy will be discussed in later sections of this paper. Yet, regardless of the particular problems with the specific approach, it is important to acknowledge the broad interest in the psychotherapeutic community in identifying and understanding the particular forms of influence that characterise psychotherapy and distinguishing these from illegitimate forms of influence on the patient. Freud's ongoing concern with the problem of suggestion, and his attempt to establish psychoanalysis as a scientific method that requires therapists to aspire to an ideal of neutrality, was one of the earliest and probably most influential approach to the question of the limits of legitimate therapeutic intervention.

From Freudian psychoanalysis onwards, the primary focus of therapists with regard to the problem of paternalism has been the problem of imposing the therapist's values on the patient. Most approaches to therapy agree that not interfering with the patient's values is a fundamental professional obligation, a broad agreement among therapies as diverse as traditional psychoanalysis and cognitive-behavioural therapy. The ethical basis that is presented for that obligation seems however, to be mixed. On the one hand it draws on the core anti-paternalist value of autonomy. It is understood that patients, as with any person, need to be free to endorse their own values and choose a way of life in accordance with it, rather than being forced or manipulated into living according to values that are not genuinely their own. Yet at the same time the justification of this demand for non-interference in therapeutic theory is also frequently presented in strongly instrumental terms: it is assumed that therapy simply would not work if it interfered with patients' values. Value neutrality, accordingly, is often addressed as a prudential rather moral obligation.

Nevertheless, it still seems fair to describe anti-paternalism as a broadly endorsed, fundamental moral obligation in the therapeutic profession. In addition to the concern of non-interference with the patient's values, anti-paternalism also manifests itself in a particular understanding of the patient's role as a moral equal in the therapeutic relationship. The importance of this attitude has increased especially since the 1960s, when the emphasis on the fundamental equality between patient and therapist not only became the object of theoretical reflection, but also became reflected in the wide-spread preference of the term "client" over "patient", which nowadays is near universal. The ethical significance of this preference for the term "client" lies in the assumption that this term highlights the contractual nature of the therapeutic relationship as a professional one between equals. Many therapists prefer this conceptualisation of the nature of the therapeutic relationship to what they consider the more clearly hierarchical relationship that "patients" find themselves in. From this viewpoint, patient status in psychotherapy implies a worrying kind of inequality insofar as the patient status in this case is based on assuming a "sickness of the mind", which can easily lead to assuming the legitimacy of their deauthorisation.

In broad terms, the assumption of non-paternalism and fundamental equality between therapist and patient goes hand in hand with the preference for therapeutic interventions of a non-directive nature. Non-directive interventions are interventions that avoid prescriptions to the patient and limit themselves to providing potential interpretations or courses of actions, with the understanding that the patient needs to be free to determine whether these are appropriate to their own situation. Therapists from the psychodynamic or humanist traditions endorse non-directivity as an essential part of their therapeutic theories. But even those therapists who, like cognitive-behavioural therapists, understand their therapeutic task as fairly directive, for example, as giving professional advice to the patient and encouraging them to work through pre-defined exercise programmes, usually encourage the patient to explore their concerns and personal attitudes to the therapist's suggestions and to accept the therapist's guidance only after conscious reflection and discussion of their concerns. As in the case of the non-interference with the patient's values, there is a certain ambiguity in the arguments that are used to support the practice of non-directive interventions, insofar as most therapists establish the need for these interventions in instrumental rather than moral terms.

This ambiguity between moral obligation and merely instrumental professional considerations will be explored further in the context of the problem of value-neutrality and will assist in the understanding of the particular way in which anti-paternalism is realised in therapy. The discussion in the following will rely on a reconceptualisation of the problem of paternalism in terms of the concepts of authority and influence. These notions provide a helpful conceptual adjustment to the particular characteristics of the therapeutic situation that help to highlight the particular ways in which paternalism manifests itself in the context of psychotherapy. This adjustment is necessary because neither the usual ethical focus on the issue of intentional deception or coercion, nor the psychotherapeutic concern with value neutrality and non-directivity are sufficiently sensitive to the particular ethical problems that therapists face in therapy. As will be shown, the notions of therapeutic authority and therapeutic influence are particularly suitable for conceptualising the problems with regard to paternalism that therapists face in the therapeutic relationship.

The notion of authority helps to conceptualise the ethical challenge that therapists face in determining what constitutes legitimate intervention. It is closely linked to the notions of autonomy and competence, both the patient's and the therapist's, but captures the particular ethical challenge that therapists face with regard to paternalism better than either of these. The notion of therapeutic influence encompasses a broad range of different modes in which the therapist's interventions may have an impact on the patient and help move the patient towards the therapist's explicit or implicit therapeutic goals. By being weaker notions than coercion or deception, notions that would imply the therapist's explicit coercive or deceptive intent, they can capture those modes of influence that are the characteristically most problematic forms of influence in therapy. What sets therapy apart from other professions in which a variety of forms of hidden influence occur, is not only the degree to which the therapists' professional practice is prone to these particular modes of influence, but especially the expectation that due to the type of their specific professional expertise, therapists achieve transparency with regard to their exercise of such influence. By approaching the problem of paternalism in therapy through this reconceptualisation, it becomes possible to explore previously hidden aspects of paternalism in that area of practice.

2. Values, Therapeutic Influence and the Scope of Therapeutic Authority

To describe a certain practice in professional contexts as paternalistic implies that this practice is not part of the scope of legitimate professional authority. The question of what practice counts as pater-nalistic presupposes an answer to the question of what kind of prob-lems and issues a professional is qualified to address authoritatively qua being a professional. Professional authority derives from the particular training that professionals undergo that equips them with particular knowledge and skills that laypersons do not possess and is limited by the scope of that particular professional knowledge. On the one hand, professional authority is limited by those areas of spe-cialist knowledge that the particular professional does not possess. Yet on the other hand, there are areas of human practice which are often considered to be outside of the boundary of any specialist pro-fessional authority. In liberal societies, there is a consensus that nobody is entitled to assume authority over what particular values people should endorse and how they should live.

Overstepping the boundaries of professional authority can there-fore either take the form of assuming specialist competence that one does not have or in mislabelling interventions as professional even though the professional should encounter the other on an equal foot-ing with regard to that specific area of concern. In most professional contexts, the second limitation of professional authority is not par-ticularly problematic insofar as potential recipients of professional services either will not look for professional advice if they consider themselves to possess sufficient competence already, or will not take such advice on board even if they are given it and they have suffi-cient confidence in their own power of judgment.

However, in the case of psychotherapy, the boundaries of what is or is not within the scope of professional competence are much more difficult to establish. In comparison with medicine, one of the fields of professional practice where problems of paternalism have been frequently addressed, determining the scope of professional compe-tence in psychotherapy is a considerably more difficult endeavour. Psychotherapy is by its very nature to a large extent concerned with how people live their lives, and it is not easy to determine how pro-fessional therapists can work with their patients on problems with regard to their personal lives without overstepping the boundaries of professional competence.

The most frequently endorsed solution to this problem in therapy is to attempt to define therapists' knowledge as purely factual and provide guidelines that will enable therapists to apply it in a value-free manner. Therapeutic expertise is thus conceptualised as purely factual specialist psychological expertise that addresses questions of psychological functioning and the mechanisms underlying the facilitation of psychological change. Based on this understanding, two popular interpretations can be distinguished regarding the value-freedom in therapeutic practice. On the one hand, as for example in cognitive behavioural therapy, the therapist's task is interpreted as being restricted to that kind of content that is psychologically objective and value-free. On this understanding, the psychologically most desirable treatment of matters of value is their psychologisation; a descriptive and presumably value-neutral interpretation in terms of psychological mechanisms. On the other hand, as for example in client-centred therapy, therapists might see their task as being independent of any content, and regard themselves only as specialists for the process of psychological change. According to this position, the therapist focuses just on the structure and framework of therapeutic interaction that is required for facilitating a constructive psychological process and is therefore not faced with the problem of values at all. On this interpretation, the therapist acts within the realm of therapeutic authority as long as he restricts his interventions to ensuring the necessary parameters of the process of change.

Yet both of these approaches to addressing the problem of value imposition in therapeutic interaction have a flaw that lies in a basic misunderstanding of the challenge they are facing: given the general task of therapeutic interaction, it is impossible to eliminate values as elements of therapeutic action. Therapeutic actions are deeply imbued with values, no matter what attempts therapists make to eliminate them from their actions. What makes the general strategy with regard to values so ethically problematic is that these attempts at elimination may in effect lead therapists to become oblivious to important aspects in which they impose their values on patients.

Why is the elimination strategy inadequate? Avoiding value content altogether or reframing any reference to values in value-neutral psychological terms might seem like a promising strategy at first sight. However, the problem lies in the subject matter of therapeutic interaction in general: it necessarily addresses the problem of how patients live their personal lives, and no matter how therapists approach the problem, whatever guidance they give to patients has relevance for the method with which these patients attempt to address their problems. Even innocuous seeming aspects of the therapeutic interaction carry implicit broader significance.

For example, ignoring patient's moral concerns when they are voiced sends a certain message to patients with regard to the importance of such considerations. When in cognitive-behavioural therapy, endorsement of binding moral norms is criticised as a failure of reasoning. This is certainly not morally neutral; this position relies on a certain understanding of the foundations and characteristics of acceptable norms in thinking. Even a therapeutic approach that neither ignores nor criticises moral concerns, but transforms them into the apparently value neutral language of psychological patterns or mechanisms, is ultimately not value neutral. Despite its seeming neutrality, it conveys to patients that addressing their problem in moral terms is a misunderstanding of what is really at issue. In shifting the focus towards the patient's own psychological functioning, the framing of the problem and the path to a possible solution is changed. Finally, even an approach that does not rephrase moral considerations as different kinds of concerns, but encourages the patient to listen to their own "inner voice", as for example in client-centred therapy, thereby proposes a certain preferable mode of solution that may very well be at odds with the patient's own preconceptions concerning moral justification. Paradoxically, the therapists' attempts to remain strictly within the area of their psychological competence may have the effect of influencing the patient in exactly the way that they profess to avoid.

The more general problem underlying the strategy of elimination is the neglect of the broader context of therapeutic interaction. The therapist's work takes place within a particular therapeutic framework that comes with a whole range of theoretical assumptions. Therapeutic theories do not just prescribe techniques of addressing psychological issues, these techniques arise from a much richer understanding of what psychological well-being consists of and how psychological problems relate to it. These broader conceptions are expressed in most of the therapist's interventions, no matter how non-directive and neutral they may appear. By means of focusing on particular types of content, therapists effectively offer a reconceptualisation of a variety of issues, for example the definition of the problem, the definition of the self, or the definition of relationships to others. Even in interactions that are not explicitly conceptual, such underlying general attitudes are effectively transmitted: through engaging patients in specific therapeutic interventions and discouraging other kinds of action, or through evoking strong positive or negative emotions, the patient undergoes a process of implicit learning about the therapist's attitudes that does not rely on the therapist's explicit expression of their underlying ideals of human development and well-being.

Therapists often seem unaware of the normative character of such ideals that underlie and define their practice. What is easily overlooked in focusing on the careful application of particular techniques is the fact that these techniques are employed to reach particular goals and that these goals are not entirely based on value-neutral psychological science, but on a broader understanding of fundamental characteristics of what should be part of a human life and imply or even explicitly outline a certain metaphysics. Therapeutic theories are not just assortments of techniques that happen to affect human life according to scientific principles; rather they are developed and employed in order to help realise a particular understanding of human life. Attempting to eliminate values from therapeutic interaction is therefore not only unachievable, but is based on a fundamental misunderstanding of the character of therapeutic practice.

3. The Therapeutic Role, Equality and Authority Shifts

If eliminating values in therapy altogether is not a viable option, how can the problem of paternalism be addressed instead? As will be proposed, therapists should consider a strategy change: rather than treat matters of values as unwelcome intrusion into therapy, they could be integrated as welcome, important constituents of the therapeutic process. Instead of, so to speak, seeing values as the enemy of therapy, to be observed with suspicion, fought and ideally eliminated, they should be regarded as potential allies of both therapist and patient that need to be attended to with respect.

The challenge in this situation is how the matter of values can be addressed without falling into paternalism. Therapists need to look for ways of interacting with the patient that enable them to integrate matters of value in their therapeutic interaction without claiming particular professional competence for them. What cannot be ignored is that therapists do engage on a daily basis with questions of the good life. Through their professional practice therapists gain extensive experience with the intimate lives of their patients and are acquainted intimately with the practical realisation of different conceptions of the good life. However, on the anti-paternalism view that is characteristic of the broadly liberal consensus of the societies in which psychotherapy is most prominent, the knowledge gained through this particular professional experience does not justify an imposition of their conclusions on their patients. While perhaps even anti-paternalists may concede that therapists are indeed in a good position to appreciate the practical realities of different realisations of the good life, this does not translate into a justification for imposing a particular value framework on unsuspecting patients who enter therapy with the expectation of receiving psychological help but not moral counsel.

One of the core assumptions of anti-paternalism is that with regard to matters of value there are no superior authorities; each individual should have the freedom, and accordingly also the responsibility, to make their own choices. Many political liberalists will argue that there is a significant distinction to be made between having the same freedom and having the same degree of authority, insofar as the freedom that the anti-paternalist protects may just be the freedom to be foolish. However, anti-paternalism in the Kantian tradition takes a stronger stance with regard to freedom and moral authority. On a Kantian understanding, the individual's freedom is based on the ability to be a fully authoritative moral agent. In a Kantian framework, all moral agents find themselves on an equal footing with regard to matters of value. While there are numerous problems with the Kantian position, the core intuition of equal moral authority resonates with many contemporaries who live in pluralist societies.

One problem of this assumption in the context of psychotherapy might be the issue of patient competence: after all, patients usually enter psychotherapy because they are experiencing problems with their psychological functioning. They look for help with regard to matters which other people manage to address independently. Would it not be fair to assume that the kind of authority that applies to fully competent persons might not apply equally to patients who suffer from psychological impairment? In this context, it needs to be kept in mind that the impairments that patients experience when they enter psychotherapy are comparatively minor with regard to their general mental competence. Unlike psychotic patients, patients who enter psychotherapy usually show satisfactory general competence with regard to most determinants of mental competence and only show impairments in some very specific fields. It would be inappropriate to assume that psychotherapy patients are generally too impaired to be taken seriously as a moral equal. The danger of overly pathologising psychotherapy patients is probably more acute than the danger of overestimating their moral competence. It is ultimately the therapist's responsibility to assess the extent and significance of patients' impairments, but it can be assumed that in most cases it will not be appropriate to consider them impaired in their general competence.

If sufficient competence for the assumption of equal moral authority can be assumed, then the relationship between therapist and patient cannot be understood as homogenous. Within the same therapeutic relationship, two very distinct types of relationship are realised: on the one hand, there is a hierarchical relationship between a psychology specialist and a patient in need of the therapist's psychological expertise; on the other hand, there is a relationship between moral equals. The challenge that therapists face is how to act on their psychological authority, with regard to which patient and therapist are unequal, without at the same time extending the same inequality to the question of moral authority, in which they do need to be considered equal.

In a relationship of such an inhomogeneous nature, authority shifts will occur during the therapeutic interaction. While in many parts of the therapeutic communication therapists will be assigned higher authority in their claims and actions due to their psychological expertise, but when matters of value are concerned, therapist and patient meet as equals. The existence of this duality within the therapeutic relationship explains why the elimination of values from therapeutic communication seems such an attractive strategy. It may seem more desirable to restrict therapeutic communication to those areas where therapists have indeed special authority, rather than finding a way of integrating specialist and non-specialist communication. However, as such elimination is not an option the responsibility for managing these authority shifts lies in the therapist's hands.

The therapist's responsibility for the management of the therapeutic interaction shifts and extends into those areas where patient and therapist encounter each other as equals. The reason why it cannot be left to the patient alone to reclaim his authority, even though this would be expected of him in ordinary circumstances, is that therapy is a form of interaction that differs in important respects from everyday interaction. The patient usually, and rightly, expects to be guided by the therapist with regard to what is appropriate behaviour in the therapeutic context. Often patients are willing to engage in actions in therapeutic contexts that they would never engage in under other circumstances. This willingness, while often constructive and in the service of therapeutic change, can sometimes be to the patient's disadvantage insofar as he might not feel entitled to make claims that they would take to be entirely appropriate under ordinary circumstances. This problem becomes even more acute given the particular insecurity and vulnerability of many patients who enter psychotherapy.

Therefore the very minimum that the therapist needs to ensure is clarification of the limits of therapeutic authority to the patient and making the shifts of authority transparent in the therapeutic interaction. The patient may be willing to relinquish authority in the service of therapeutic progress; the therapist's responsibility is to make sure that this does not occur with regard to those aspects where the therapist encounters the patient on an equal footing. The main assumption underlying the demand for transparency is that the transparency of the therapist's values may be more effectively anti-paternalistic than any attempt to "neutralise" therapeutic action, insofar as the latter will often do more to disguise the value-laden nature of the action and thereby disempower the patient. Explicating values enables the patient to engage with his own views and the therapist's suggestions as matters of value and not as professional expertise to which he can be expected to defer.

4. The Moral Weight of Implicit Therapeutic Influence

In view of the comparatively subtle manifestations of therapeutic authority that were outlined above, the question may arise of whether it is appropriate at all to consider these as constituting paternalism. After all, such forms of influence are ubiquitous, not just in all kinds of professional relationships, but in any kind of human interaction. If hidden and implicit forms of influence are included, even if they do not involve a clearly identifiable act of coercion or deception on the part of the agent, the danger is that it becomes impossible to draw a line between paternalistic interventions and forms of influence that are morally legitimate, if somewhat undesirable and problematic. Should the use of the term "paternalism" not be restricted to a more limited class of actions, namely those where more explicit and drastic infringements of a person's autonomy are concerned?

While this is a legitimate concern, the main goal in this context lies in establishing the reasons for giving a similar *moral weight* to certain forms of psychotherapeutic influence as is usually given to more paradigmatic forms of paternalism. Whether or not such action should be given the label "paternalism" will be left open for the time being. The term paternalism has been used so far in order to draw attention to the moral similarities between paternalistic action and certain aspects of therapeutic action. What is at issue here is the family resemblance between this form of therapeutic influence and paternalism; whether it should ultimately be regarded as identical twin or just as the cousin of paternalistic action will be left open for the time being.

What gives hidden therapeutic influence this particular moral significance? The implicit forms of influence that are characteristic of therapeutic interaction affect many forms of communication. The problem of professional influence arises in all professional relationships, due to the hierarchical nature of a relationship in which the professional has expertise that the client does not have. Professionals in most specialties have a significant influence on the client's perception of what constitutes a good solution to their problem merely by presenting the "facts" in certain ways. However, in the case of psychotherapy such influence constitutes a particularly significant moral issue because of the particular characteristics of the therapeutic role. Whereas in other professional relationships the communication between professional and client is, in a sense, a prelude to the proper exercise of the professional's specialist knowledge, in therapy this communication is what constitutes the very application of the specialist knowledge. Being such a specialist increases the therapist's responsibility in comparison to other professionals: unlike other professionals, for therapists it is part of the therapeutic role to be attentive to implicit aspects of communication and to effectively control their exercise.

More than other professionals, therapists' professionalism is expected to ensure a self-transparent exercise of their expertise. What makes this responsibility especially significant is the fact that patients usually seek psychotherapy because of problems that make them potentially more vulnerable than clients in other kinds of professional relationships. Establishing a working therapeutic relationship often requires a degree of emotional intensity that makes questioning or giving up such a relationship much more difficult than would be the case for other kinds of professional relationships. Due to the nature of their problems patients may also feel less confident of their own perceptions and more likely to accept what therapists suggest to them. In a relationship that involves these ingredients, the impact of implicit forms of influence can be assumed to be not just potentially stronger, but also potentially more significant than in many other professional or human interactions. What is at issue in therapy is often a re-examination of the very foundations of the patient's life; professional interventions that address this problem can have an impact that the patient may not be able to control. It therefore seems legitimate to apply standards to therapeutic interaction that do not apply to members in other professions. Due to the particular features of the therapeutic situation, hidden forms of influence in psychotherapy have a moral significance that greatly exceed the significance of similar actions in different contexts and justifies addressing it in the context of paternalism.

PERSONALIA

George Agich is professor at the Department of Philosophy of Bowling Green State University in Ohio and Director of the BGeXperience Program.

His publications include: *Dependence and Autonomy in Old Age. An Ethical Framework for Long-Term Care*, Cambridge University Press, 2003; 'Autonomy and the Ethics of Neurosurgery,' (with E. Mordini) in *Italian Journal of Psychiatry and Behavioural Sciences* 2(1998); 'Can the Patient Make Treatment Decisions? Evaluationg Decisional Capacities' in *Cleveland Clinic Journal of Medicine* 64(1997)9; 'Disease, Functions, Values, and Psychiatric Classification,' (with J. Sadler) in *Philosophy, Psychiatry, and Psychology*, 2(1995); 'Key Concepts: Autonomy,' in *Philosophy, Psychiatry, and Psychology* 1(1994); *Autonomy and Long-Term Care*, Oxford University Press, 1993; *Responsibility in Health Care*, Reidel Publishing, 1982.

David Archard is Professor of Philosophy and Public Policy and Director of the Institute of Environment, Philosophy & Public Policy at Lancaster University.

His recent publications include *Sexual Consent*, Westview, 1998; *Children, Rights and Childhood*, Routledge, 1993, 2nd edition forthcoming in 2004; *Children, Family and State*, Ashgate, 2003; and the co-edited with Colin Macleod, *The Moral and Political Status of Children*, Oxford University Press, 2002. He has numerous articles and chapters in moral, political and legal philosophy. Just published is 'Wrongful Life' in *Philosophy* and 'Political Reasonableness' is forthcoming in *Canadian Journal of Philosophy*.

Yvonne Denier, Ph.D., is Research Fund K.U.Leuven post-doctoral researcher in moral philosophy at the Faculty of Philosophy and at the Faculty of Economics of the Catholic University of Leuven, Belgium.

She is author of *Efficiency, Justice and Care. Philosophical Reflections on Scarcity in Health Care* (Springer, 2007, forthcoming), of 'Need or Desire? A Conceptual and Moral Phenomenology of the Child Wish' (in *International Journal of Applied Philosophy* 20(2006)1), and of 'On Personal Responsibility & the Human Right to Health Care' (*Cambridge Quarterly of Healthcare Ethics* 14(2005)2).

Eva Kittay, is Professor of Philosophy at the State University of New York at Stony Brook.

Her publications include *The Subject of Care: Feminist Perspectives on Dependency* (with Ellen Feder) Rowman and Littlefield, 2002; 'Can Contractualism

Justify State-Supported Long-Term Care Policies?' in *World Health Organisation*, 2002; 'Caring for the Vulnerable by Caring for the Caregiver: The Case of Mental Retardation,' in R. Rhodes et al. (eds), *Health Care and Distributive Justice*, Oxford University Press, 2002; 'When Care is Just and Justice is Caring: The Case of the Care for the Mentally Retarded,' in *Public Culture* 13(2001)3; 'From Welfare from a Public Ethics of Care,' in N. Hirschmann et al. (eds.), *Women and Welfare*, Rutgers University Press, 2001; *Love's Labor: Essays on Women, Equality, and Dependency*, Routledge 1999.

Eric Matthews is Emeritus Professor of Philosophy and Honorary Research Professor of Medical and Psychiatric Ethics in the University of Aberdeen, Scotland.

Recent publications include: 'Mental and Physical Illness: An Unsustainable Separation?' in Eastman and Peay (eds), *Law without Enforcement*, Hart Publishing, 1999; 'Autonomy and the Psychiatric Patient,' *Journal of Applied Philosophy*, 17(2000)1; 'Personal Identity and Mental Health,' in Thomasma, Weisstub and Hervé (eds), *Personhood and Health Care*, Kluwer, 2001; 'How can a mind be sick?, in Fullford, Sadler and Stanghellini (eds), *Nature and Narrative*, Oxford University Press, 2003; 'Merleau-Ponty's Body-Subject and Psychiatry,' *International Review of Psychiatry*, 16, 2004.

Thomas Nys, Ph.D., is post-doctoral researcher in moral philosophy at the Centre for Ethics of the Catholic University of Leuven.

Recent publications include: 'Re-sourcing the Self? Isaiah Berlin and Charles Taylor: The Tension between Freedom and Authenticity', in *Ethical Perspectives* 11(2004)4; 'Psychiatry under Pressure: Reflections on Psychiatry's Drift Towards a Reductionist Biomedical Conception of Mental Illness' in *Medicine, Health Care and Philosophy* 9(2006)1; 'Paternalisme en autonomie in de geestelijke gezondheidszorg' [Paternalism and Autonomy in Mental Health Care] in *Tijdschrift voor Psychiatrie*, 47(2005)8; 'On Suicide and Other Comforts' in Neumaier, Sedmark & Zichy (eds.), *Philosophische Perspektiven. Beiträge zum VII. Internationalen Kongress der ÖGP* (2005), Lancaster, Ontos.

Heike Schmidt-Felzmann, Ph.D., is Lecturer in Philosophy at the National University of Ireland, Galway, and Co-Director of the Centre of Bioethical Research and Analysis.

Recent publications include: 'Pragmatic Principles: Methodological Pragmatism in Biomedical Ethics,' in: *The Journal of Medicine and Philosophy* 28(2003)5-6; 'Gegenwärtige Vergangenheit und vergängliche Gegenwart? Erinnern in der Psychoanalyse' in: Ch. Lotz, T. Wolf, W. Zimmerli (eds.): *Erinnerung — Philosophische Positionen und Perspektiven*, Wilhelm Fink, 2004; ‚Neuroethik — Zum Zusammenhang zwischen Neurowissenschaft und Ethik,' Ausgewählte Beiträge der GAP5, 2004

Toon Vandevelde is Professor of Philosophy at the Faculty of Philosophy and at the Faculty of Economics of the Catholic University of Leuven, Belgium.

He is author of numerous articles, books, and chapters in moral, social and political philosophy. His publications include 'Participation, Immortality and the Gift Economy: An Introduction to the Work of Burkhard Sievers,' in *Ethical Perspectives* 3(1996)3; *Is Inheritance Legitimate?* (with G. Erreygers), Springer, 1997; *Gifts and Interests* (ed.), Peeters, 2000; 'Ethical Aspects of Debt Reduction for the Poorest Countries' (with J. Van Gerwen) in *Ethical Perspectives* 8(2001)1; 'The Ethics of Sex Selection for Non-Medical Reasons' (with B. Engelen) in *Ethical Perspectives* 11(2004)1; Just published are 'Beyond Liberalism?' in *Frontline* 22(2005)4 and 'What Do We Owe the World's Poor?' in *Ethical Perspectives* 12(2005)4.

PRINTED ON PERMANENT PAPER • IMPRIME SUR PAPIER PERMANENT • GEDRUKT OP DUURZAAM PAPIER - ISO 9706

N.V. PEETERS S.A., WAROTSTRAAT 50, B-3020 HERENT